AF659959

Hospital Rules and Regulations

Hospital Rules and Regulations

C.Charles

ANMOL PUBLICATIONS PVT. LTD.
NEW DELHI - 110 002 (INDIA)

ANMOL PUBLICATIONS PVT. LTD.
H.O.: 4374/4B, Ansari Road, Darya Ganj
New Delhi-110 002 (India)
Ph.: 23278000, 23261597
B.O.: 1015, Ist Main Road, BSK IIIrd Stage
IIIrd Phase, IIIrd Block
Bangalore - 560 085 (Karnataka)
Ph: 080-41723429, Tel/Fax: 080-2672 3604
Visit us at: www.anmolpublications.com

Hospital Rules and Regulations

© Reserved

First Published, 2008

ISBN 978-81-261-3286-7

PRINTED IN INDIA

Printed at Mehra Offset Press, Delhi.

Contents

Contents

Preface

This book titled "Hospital Rules and Regulations" deals with the international and national guidelines related to hospitals in India and abroad.

This book contains details regarding Medical Acts, Rules and Regulations in India; Rules for Hospital and Health Services; Regulations for Hospital and Diagnostic Centres; Guidelines for Nursing Home and Medical Devices Administration; Health Authorities Acts and Rules; Hospital and Health Insurance Acts; Health Care Laws; Public Health Acts, Guidelines and Ethics; Competition Laws for Hospitals, Physicians and Pharmaceutical etc.

This book titled "Hospital Rules and Regulations" is of great contemporary relevance as far as hospital administration and management is concerned worldwide, including India. It also critically analyses the recent moves of the central and state governments to enact hospital and nursing home laws in various states of India to regulate the medical practices. Besides, it reflects on major global scenario in this regard.

—Editor

1

Medical Acts, Rules and Regulations in India

THE INDIAN MEDICAL COUNCIL ACT, 1956
(102 of 1956)

30th December, 1956
(As amended by the Indian Medical Council (Amendment) Acts, 1964, 1993 & 2001)

AN ACT TO PROVIDE FOR THE RECONSTITUTION OF THE MEDICAL COUNCIL OF INDIA AND THE MAINTENANCE OF A MEDICAL REGISTER FOR INDIA AND FOR MATTERS CONNECTED THEREWITH.

Be it enacted by Parliament in the seventh year of the Republic of India as follows:-

Short Title, Extent and Commencement

1.

1. This Act may be called the Indian Medical Council Act, 1956.
2. It extends to the whole of India.
3. It shall come into force on such date as the Central Government may, by notification in the Official Gazette, appoint.

Definitions

2. In this Act, unless the context otherwise requires:-

(a) "approved institution" means a hospital, health centre or other such institution recognised

(b) by a university as an institution in which a person may undergo the training, if any, required by his course of study before the award of any medical qualification to him.

(c) "council" means the Medical Council of India constituted under this Act.

(d) ["deleted" by Indian Medical Council (Amendment) Act, 1964.]

(e) "Indian Medical Register" means the medical register maintained by the Council.

(f) "Medical Institution" means any institution, within or without India, which grants degrees, diplomas or licences in medicine.

(g) "medicine" means modern scientific medicine in all its branches and includes surgery and obstetrics, but does not include veterinary medicine and surgery;

(h) "Prescribed" means prescribed by regulations.

(i) "recognised medical qualification" means any of the medical qualifications included in the Schedules.

(j) "regulation" means a regulation made under section 33;

(k) "State Medical Council" means a medical council constituted under any law for the time being in force in any State regulating the registration of practitioners of medicine.

(l) "State Medical Register" means a register maintained under any law for the time being in force in any State regulating the registration of practitioners of medicine.

(m) "University" means any University in India established by law and having a medical faculty.

Constitution and Composition of the Council

3.

1. The Central Government shall cause to be constituted a council consisting of the following members, namely:-

   (a) One member from each State other than a Union Territory to be nominated by the Central Government in consultation with the State Government concerned.

   (b) One member from each University to be elected from amongst the members of the medical faculty of the University by members of the Senate of the University or in case the University has no Senate, by members of the Court.

   (c) One member from each State in which a State Medical Register is maintained, to be elected from amongst themselves by persons enrolled on such register who possess the medical qualifications included in the First or the Second Schedule or in Part II of the Third Schedule.

   (d) Seven members to be elected from amongst themselves by persons enrolled on any of the State Medical Registers who possess the medical qualifications included in Part I of the Third Schedule.

(e) Eight members to be nominated by the Central Govt.

2. The President and Vice-President of the Council shall be elected by the members of the Council from amongst themselves.

3. No act done by the Council shall be questioned on the ground merely of the existence of any vacancy in, or any defect in the constitution of the Council.

Mode of Election

4.

1. (a) An election under clause (b), clause (c) or clause (d) of sub-section (1) of section 3 shall be conducted by the Central Government in accordance with such rules as may be made by it in this behalf, and any rules so made may provide that pending the preparation of the Indian Medical Register in accordance with provisions of this Act, the members referred to in clause (d) of sub-section (1) of section 3 may be nominated by the Central Government instead of being elected as provided therein.

2. Where any dispute arises regarding any election to the Council, it shall be referred to the Central Government whose decision shall be final.

Restrictions on Nomination and Membership

5.

1. No person shall be eligible for nomination under clause (a) of sub-section (1) of section 3 unless he possesses any of the medical qualifications included in the First and Second Schedules, resides in the State concerned, and where a State Medical Register is maintained in that State, is enrolled on that Register.

2. No person may at the same time serve as a member in more than one capacity.

Incorporation of the Council

6.

The Council so constituted shall be a body corporate by the name of the Medical Council of India, having perpetual succession and a common seal, with power to acquire and hold property, both movable and immovable, and to contract and shall by the said name sue and be sued.

Term of Office of President, Vice-president and Members

7.

1. The President or Vice-President of the Council shall hold office for a term not exceeding five years and not extending beyond the expiry of his term as member of the Council.
2. Subject to the provisions of this section, a member shall hold office for a term of five years from the date of his nomination or election or until his successor shall have been duly nominated or elected, whichever is longer.
3. An elected or nominated member shall be deemed to have vacated his seat if he is absent without excuse, sufficient in the opinion of the Council from three consecutive ordinary meetings of the Council, or in the case of a member elected under clause (b) of sub-section (1) of section 3, if he ceases to be a member of the medical faculty of the university concerned, or in the case of a member elected under clause (c) or clause (d) of that sub-section, if he ceases to be a person enrolled on the State Medical Register concerned.
4. A casual vacancy in the Council shall be filled by

nomination or election, as the case may be, and the person nominated or elected to fill the vacancy shall hold office only for the remainder of the term for which the member whose place he takes was nominated or elected.

5. Members of the Council shall be eligible for re-nomination or re-election.
6. Where the said term of five years is about to expire in respect of any member, a successor may be nominated or elected at any time within three months before the said term expires but he shall not assume office until the said term has expired.

Meetings of the Council

8.

1. The Council shall meet at least once in each year at such time and place as may be appointed by the Council.
2. Unless otherwise provided by regulations fifteen members of the Council shall form a quorum, and all the acts of the Council shall be decided by a majority of the members present and voting.

Officers, Committees and Servants of the Council

9. The Council Shall:

1. constitute from amongst its members an Executive Committee and such other committees for general or special purposes as the Council deems necessary to carry out the purposes of this Act.
2. appoint a Registrar who shall act as Secretary and who may also, if deemed expedient, act as Treasurer.
3. employ such other persons, as the Council deems necessary to carry out the purposes of this Act.

4. require and take from the Registrar, or from any other employee, such security for the due performance of his duties as the Council deems necessary and
5. With the previous sanction of the Central Government fix the remuneration and allowances to be paid to the President, Vice-President and members of the Council and determine the conditions of service of the employees of the Council.

The Executive Committee

10.

1. The Executive Committee, hereinafter referred to as the Committee shall consist of the President and Vice-President, who shall be members ex-officio and not less than seven and not more than ten other members who shall be elected by the Council from amongst its members.
2. The President and Vice-President shall be the President and Vice-President respectively of the Committee.
3. In addition to the powers and duties conferred and imposed upon it by this Act, the Committee shall exercise and discharge such powers and duties as the Council may confer or impose upon it by any regulations which may be made in this behalf.

Permission for Establishment of New Medical College, New Course of Study etc.

10.A

1. Notwithstanding anything contained in this Act or any other law for the time being in force:-
   (a) no person shall establish a medical colleg
   (or)

(b) no medical college shall:-

(i) open a new or higher course of study or training (including a postgraduate course of study or training) which would enable a student of such course or training to qualify himself for the award of any recognised medical qualification; or

(ii) increase its admission capacity in any course of study or training (including a postgraduate course of study or training), except with the previous permission of the Central Government obtained in accordance with the provisions of this section.

Explanation 1 - For the purposes of this section, "person" includes any University or a trust but does not include the Central Government.

Explanation 2 - For the purposes of this section "admission capacity" in relation to any course of study or training (including postgraduate course of study or training) in a medical college, means the maximum number of students that may be fixed by the Council from time to time for being admitted to such course or training.

2.

(a) Every person or medical college shall, for the purpose of obtaining permission under sub-section (1), submit to the Central Government a scheme in accordance with the provisions of clause (b) and the central Government shall refer the scheme to the Council for its recommendations.

(b) The Scheme referred to in clause (a) shall be in such form and contain such particulars and be preferred in such manner and be accompanied with such fee as may be prescribed.

3. On receipt of a scheme by the Council under sub-section (2) the Council may obtain such other particulars as may be considered necessary by it from the person or the medical college concerned, and thereafter, it may -
   (a) if the scheme is defective and does not contain any necessary particulars, give a reasonable opportunity to the person or college concerned for making a written representation and it shall be open to such person or medical college to rectify the defects, if any, specified by the Council.
   (b) consider the scheme, having regard to the factors referred to in sub-section (7) and submit the scheme together with its recommendations thereon to the Central Government.
4. The Central Govt. may after considering the scheme and the recommendations of the Council under sub-section (3) and after obtaining, where necessary, such other particulars as may be considered necessary by it from the person or college concerned, and having regard to the factors referred to in sub-section (7), either approve (with such conditions, if any, as it may consider necessary) or disapprove the scheme, and any such approval shall be a permission under sub-section (1):

Provided that no scheme shall be disapproved by the Central Government except after giving the person or college concerned a reasonable opportunity of being heard; Provided further that nothing in this sub section shall prevent any person or medical college whose scheme has not been approved by the Central Government to submit a fresh scheme and the provisions of this section shall apply to such scheme, as if such scheme has been submitted for the first time under sub-section (1).

5. Where, within a period of one year from the date of submission of the scheme to the Central Government under sub-section (1), no order passed by the Central Government has been communicated to the person or college submitting the scheme, such scheme shall be deemed to have been approved by the Central Government in the form in which it had been submitted, and accordingly, the permission of the Central Government required under sub-section (1) shall also be deemed to have been granted.
6. In computing the time-limit specified in sub-section (5), the time taken by the person or college concerned submitting the scheme, in furnishing any particulars called for by the Council, or by the Central Government, shall be excluded.
7. The Council, while making its recommendations under clause (b) of sub-section (3) and the Central Government, while passing an order, either approving or disapproving the scheme under sub-section (4), shall have due regard to the following factors, namely:-
   (a) whether the proposed medical college or the existing medical college seeking to open a new or higher course of study or training, would be in a position to offer the minimum standards of medical education as prescribed by the Council under section 19A or, as the case may be under section 20 in the case of postgraduate medical education.

(b) whether the person seeking to establish a medical college or the existing medical college seeking to open a new or higher course of study or training or to increase it admission capacity has adequate financial resources;

(c) whether necessary facilities in respect of staff, equipment, accommodation, training and other facilities to ensure proper functioning of the medical college or conducting the new course or study or training or accommodating the increased admission capacity, have been provided or would be provided within the time-limit specified in the scheme.

(d) whether adequate hospital facilities, having regard to the number or students likely to attend such medical college or course of study or training or as a result of the increased admission capacity, have been provided or would be provided within the time-limit specified in the scheme;

(e) whether any arrangement has been made or programme drawn to impart proper training to students likely to attend such medical college or course of study or training by persons having the recognised medical qualifications;

(f) the requirement of manpower in the field of practice of medicine; and any other factors as may be prescribed.

(g) Where the Central Government passes an order either approving or disapproving a scheme under this section, a copy of the order shall be communicated to the person or college concerned.

Non-Recognition of Medical Qualifications in Certain Cases

10B

1. Where any medical college is established except with the previous permission of the Central Government in accordance with the provisions of section 10A, no medical qualification granted to any student of such medical college shall a recognised medical qualification for the purposes of this Act.
2. Where any medical college opens a new or higher course of study or training (including a postgraduate course of study or training) except with the previous permission of the Central Government in accordance with the provisions of section 10A, no medical qualification granted to any student of such medical college on the basis of such study or training shall be a recognised medical qualification for the purposes of this Act.
3. Where any medical college increases its admission capacity in any course of study or training except with the previous permission of the Central Government in accordance with the provisions of section 10A, no medical qualification granted to any student of such medical college on the basis of the increase in its admission capacity shall be a recognised medical qualification for the purposes of this Act.

Explanation - For the purposes of this section, the criteria for identifying a student who has been granted a medical qualification on the basis of such increase in the admission capacity shall be such as may be prescribed.

Time for Seeking Permission for Certain Existing Medical Colleges, etc.

10C.

1. If, after, the 1st day of June, 1992 and on and before the commencement of the Indian Medical Council (Amendment) Act, 1993 any person has established a medical college or any medical college has opened a new or higher course of study or training or increased the admission capacity, such person or medical college, as the case may be, shall seek, within a period of one year from the commencement of the Indian Medical Council (Amendment) Act, 1993 the permission of the Central Government in accordance with the provisions of section 10A.
2. If any person or medical college, as the case may be fails to seek the permission under sub section (1) the provisions of section 10B shall apply, so far as may be as if, permission of the Central Government under section 10A has been refused;

Recognition of Medical Qualification Granted by Universities or Medical Institutions In India

11.

1. The medical qualifications granted by any university or medical Institution in India which are included in the first Schedule shall be recognised medical qualifications for the purposes of this Act.
2. Any university or medical Institution in India which grants a medical qualification not included in the First Schedule may apply to the Central Govt., to have such qualification recognised, and the Central Government, after consulting the Council, may, by notification in the official Gazette, amend the First Schedule so as to include such qualification therein, and any such notification may also direct that an entry shall be made in the last column of the First

Schedule against such medical qualification declaring that it shall be a recognised medical qualification only when granted after a specified date.

Recognition of Medical Qualifications Granted by Medical Institutions in Countries with which there is a Scheme of Reciprocity

12.

1. The medical qualifications granted by medical institutions outside India which are included in the Second Schedule shall be recognised medical qualifications for the purposes of this Act.
2. The Council may enter into negotiations with the Authority in any country outside India which by the law of such country is entrusted with the maintenance of a register of medical practitioners, for the settling of a scheme of reciprocity for the recognition of medical qualifications and in pursuance of any such scheme, the Central Government may, by notification in the official Gazette, amend the Second Schedule so as to include therein the medical qualification which the Council has decided should be recognised and any such notification may also direct that an entry shall be made in the last column of the Second Schedule against such medical qualification declaring that it shall be a recognised medical qualification only when granted after a specified date.
3. The Central Government, after consultation with the Council, may, by notification in the Official Gazette, amend the Second Schedule by directing that an entry be made therein in respect of any medical qualification declaring that it shall be recognised medical qualification only when granted before a specified date.

4. Where the Council has refused to recommend any medical qualification which has been proposed for recognition by any Authority referred to in sub-section (2) and that Authority applies to the Central Government in this behalf, the Central Government, after considering such application and after obtaining from the council a report, if any, as to the reasons for any such refusal, may by notification in the Official Gazette, amend the Second Schedule so as to include such qualification therein and the provisions of sub-section (2) shall apply to such notification.

Recognition of Medical Qualification Granted by Certain Medical Institutions Whose Qualifications are Not Included in the First or Second Schedule

13.

1. The medical qualifications granted by medical institutions in India which are not included in the First Schedule and which are included in Part I of the Third Schedule shall also be recognised medical qualifications for the purposes of this Act.
2. The medical qualifications granted to a citizen of India:-
   (a) before the 15th day of August, 1947, by medical institutions in the territories now forming part of Pakistan, and,
   (b) before the 1st day of April, 1937, by medical institutions in the territories now forming part of Burma, which are included in part 1 of the Third Schedule shall also be recognised medical qualifications for the purposes of this Act.
3. The medical qualifications granted by medical institutions outside India, before such date as the

Central Government may, by notification in the Official Gazette, specify which are included in Part IInd of the Third Schedule shall also be recognised medical qualifications for the purposes of this Act, but no person possessing any such qualification shall be entitled to enrolment on any State Medical Register unless he is a citizen of India and has undergone such practical training after obtaining that qualification as may be required by the rules or regulations in force in the country granting the qualification, or if he has not undergone any practical training in that country he has undergone such practical training as may be prescribed.

4. The Central Government, after consulting the Council, may, by notification in the Official Gazette, amend Part II of the Third Schedule so as to include therein any qualification granted by a medical institution outside India, which is not included in the Second Schedule.

Provided that after the commencement of the Indian Medical Council (Amendment) Act, 2001, no such amendment shall be made in Part II of the Third Schedule to include any primary medical qualification granted by any medical institution outside India: Provided further that nothing contained in the first proviso shall apply to inclusion in Part II of the Third Schedule any primary medical qualification granted by any medical institution outside India to any person whose name is entered in the Indian Medical Register. Explanation- For the purposes of this sub-section, "primary medical qualification" means any minimum qualification sufficient for enrolment on any State Medical Register or for entering the name in the Indian Medical Register.

(4A) A person who is a citizen of India and obtains medical qualification granted by any medical institution in any country outside India recognised for enrolment as medical practitioner in that country after such date as may be specified by the Central Government under sub-section (3), shall not be entitled to be enrolled on any Medical Register maintained by a State Medical Council or to have his name entered in the Indian Medical Register unless he qualified the screening test in India prescribed for such purpose and such foreign medical qualification after such person qualifies that said screening test shall be deemed to be the recognised medical qualification for the purposes of this Act for that person.

(4B) A person who is a citizen of India shall not, after such date as may be specified by the Central Government under sub-section (3), be eligible to get admission to obtain medical qualification granted by any medical institution in any foreign country without obtaining an eligibility certificate issued to him by the Council and in case any such person obtains such qualification without obtaining such eligibility certificate, he shall not be eligible to appear in the screening test referred to in sub-section (4A):

Provided that an Indian citizen who has acquired the medical qualification from foreign medical institution or has obtained admission in foreign medical institution before the commencement of the Indian Medical Council (Amendment) Act, 2001 shall not be required to obtain eligibility certificate under this sub-section but, if he is qualified for admission to any medical course for recognised medical qualification in any medical institution in India, he shall be required to qualify only the screening test prescribed for enrolment on any State Medical Register or for entering his name in the Indian Medical Register.

(4C) Nothing contained in sub-sections (4A) and (4B) shall apply to the medical qualifications referred to in section 14 for the purposes of that section.

5. Any medical institution in India which is desirous of getting a medical qualification granted by it included in Part I of the Third Schedule may apply to the Central Government to have such qualification recognised and the Central Government, after consulting the Council, may by notification in the Official Gazette, amend Part I of the Third Schedule so as to include such qualification therein, and any such notification may also direct that an entry shall be made in the last column of Part-I of the Third Schedule against such medical qualification declaring that it shall be a recognised medical qualification only when granted after a specified date.

Special Provision In Certain Cases for Recognition of Medical Qualifications Granted by Medical Institutions in Countries with which there is no Scheme of Reciprocity

14.

1. The Central Government after consultation with the Council, may, by notification in the Official Gazette, direct that medical qualifications granted by medical institutions in any country out-side India in respect of which a scheme of reciprocity for the recognition of medical qualifications is not in force, shall be recognised medical qualification for the purposes of this Act or shall be so only when granted after a specified date:

Provided that medical practice by persons possessing such qualifications: -

(a) shall be permitted only if such persons are

enrolled as medical practitioners in accordance with the law regulating the registration of medical practitioners for the time being in force in that country;

(b) shall be limited to the institution to which they are attached for the time being for the purposes of teaching, research or charitable work ; and

(c) shall be limited to the period specified in this behalf by the Central Government by general or special order.

2. In respect of any such medical qualification the Central Government, after consultation with the Council may, by notification in the Official Gazette direct that it shall be a recognised medical qualification only when granted before a specified date.

Right of Persons Possessing Qualifications in the Schedules to be Enrolled

15.

1. Subject to the other provisions contained in this Act, the medical qualifications included in the Schedules shall be sufficient qualification for enrolment on any State Medical Register.
2. Save as provided in section 25, no person other than a medical practitioner enrolled on a State Medical Register:-

   (a) shall hold office as physician or surgeon or any other office (by whatever designation called) in Government or in any institution maintained by a local or other authority;

   (b) shall practice medicine in any State;

(c) shall be entitled to sign or authenticate a medical or fitness certificate or any other certificate required by any law to be signed or authenticated by a duly qualified medical practitioner:

(d) shall be entitled to give evidence at any inquest or in any court of law as an expert under section 45 of the Indian Evidence Act, 1872 on any matter relating to medicine.

3. Any person who acts in contravention of any provision of sub-section (2) shall be punished with imprisonment for a term which may extend to one year or with fine which may extend to one thousand rupees, or with both.

Power to Require Information as to Courses of Study and Examinations

16.

Every University or medical institution in India which grants a recognised medical qualification shall furnish such information as the Council may, from time to time, require as to the courses of study and examinations to be undergone in order to obtain such qualification, as to the ages at which such courses of study and examinations are required to be undergone and such qualification is conferred and generally as to the requisites for obtaining such qualification.

Inspection of Examinations

17.

1. The Committee shall appoint such number of medical inspectors as it may deem requisite to inspect any medical institution, college, hospital or other institution where medical education is given, or to attend any examination held by any University or

medical institution for the propose of recommending to the Central Government recognition of medical qualifications granted by the University or medical institution.

2. The medical inspectors shall not interfere with the conduct of any training or examination, but shall report to the committee on the adequacy of the standards of medical education including staff, equipment, accommodation, training facilities prescribed for giving medical education or on the sufficiency of every examination which they attend.
3. The Committee shall forward a copy of any such report to the university or medical institution concerned and shall also forward a copy with the remarks of the University or institution thereon, to the Central Government.

Visitors at Examinations

18.

1. The Council may appoint such number of visitors as it may deem requisite to inspect any medical institution, college, hospital or other institution where medical education is given, or to attend any examination held by any University or medical institution for the purpose of granting recognised medical qualifications.
2. Any person, whether he is a member of the Council or not may be appointed as a visitor under this section but a person who is appointed as an inspector under section 17 for any inspection or examination shall not be appointed as a visitor for the same inspection or examination.
3. The visitors shall not interfere with the conduct of

any training or examination but shall report to the President of the Council on the adequacy of the standards of medical education including staff, equipment, accommodation, training and other facilities prescribed for giving medical education or on the sufficiency of every examination which they attend.

4. The report of a visitor shall be treated as confidential unless in any particular case the President of the Council otherwise directs:

   Provided that if the Central Government requires a copy of the report of a visitor, the Council shall furnish the same.

Withdrawal of Recognision

19.

1. When upon report by the Committee or the visitor it appear to the Council:-
   (a) that the courses of study and examination to be undergone in, or the proficiency required from candidates at any examination held by any University or medical institution,
   (b) that the staff, equipment accommodation, training and other facilities for instruction and training provided in such University or medical institution or in any college or other institution affiliated to that University, do not conform to the standards prescribed by the Council, the Council shall make a representation to that effect to the Central Government.
2. After considering such representation, the Central Govt. may send it to the State Government of the State in which the University or medical Institution

is situated and the State Government shall forward it along with such remarks as it may choose to make to the University or Medical Institution, with an intimation of the period within which the University or medical institution may submit its explanation to the State Government.

3. On the receipt of the explanation or, where no explanation is submitted within the period fixed, then on the expiry of that period, the State Government shall make its recommendations to the Central Government
4. The Central Government, after making such further inquiry, if any, as it may think fit, may by notification in the official Gazette, direct that an entry shall be made in the appropriate Schedule against the said medical qualification declaring that it shall be a recognised medical qualification, only when granted before a specified date or that the said medical qualification if granted to students of a specified college or institution affiliated to any university shall be a recognised medical qualification only when granted before a specified date or, as the case may be, that the said medical qualification shall be a recognised medical qualification in relation to a specified college or institution affiliated to any University only when granted after a specified date.

Minimum Standards of Medical Education

19.A

1. The Council may prescribe the minimum standards of medical education required for granting recognised medical qualifications (other than postgraduate medical qualifications) by universities or medical institutions in India.

2. Copies of the draft regulations and of all subsequent amendments thereof shall be furnished by the Council to all State Governments and the Council shall before submitting the regulations or any amendment thereof, as the case may be, to the Central Government for sanction, take into consideration the comments of any State Government received within three months from the furnishing of the copies as aforesaid.
3. The Committee shall from time to time report to the Council on the efficacy of the regulations and may recommend to the Council such amendments thereof as it may think fit.

Post-graduate Medical Education Committee for Assisting Council in Matters Relating to Post-graduate Medical Education

20.

1. The Council may prescribe standards of Postgraduate Medical Education for the guidance of Universities, and may advise Universities in the matter of securing uniform standards for Postgraduate Medical Education through out India, and for this purpose the Central Govt. may constitute from among the members of the Council a Postgraduate Medical Education Committee (hereinafter referred to as the Post-graduate Committee)
2. The Postgraduate Committee shall consist of nine members all of whom shall be persons possessing postgraduate medical qualifications and experience of teaching or examining postgraduate students of medicine.
3. Six of the members of the Postgraduate Committee shall be nominated by the Central Government and the remaining three members shall be elected by

the Council from amongst its members.

4. For the purpose of considering postgraduate studies in a subject, the Postgraduate Committee may co-opt, as and when necessary, one or more members qualified to assist it in that subject.
5. The views and recommendations of the Postgraduate Committee on all matters shall be placed before the Council and if the Council does not agree with the views expressed or the recommendations made by the Postgraduate Committee on any matter, the Council shall forward them together with its observations to the Central Government for decision.

Professional Conduct

20.A

1. The Council may prescribe standards of professional conduct and etiquette and a code of ethics for medical practitioners.
2. Regulations made by the Council under sub-section (1) may specify which violations thereof shall constitute infamous conduct in any professional respect, that is to say, professional misconduct, and such provisions shall have effect notwithstanding anything contained in any law for the time being in force.

Indian Medical Register

21.

1. The Council shall cause to be maintained in the prescribed manner a register of medical practitioners to be known as the Indian Medical Register, which shall contain the names of all persons who are for the time being enrolled on any State Medical Register

and who possess any of the recognised medical qualifications.

2. It shall be the duty of the Registrar of the Council to keep the Indian Medical Register in accordance with the provisions of this Act and of any orders made by the Council, and from time to time to revise the register and publish it in the Gazette of India and in such other manner as may be prescribed.
3. Such register shall be deemed to be public document within the meaning of the Indian Evidence Act, 1872 and may be proved by a copy published in the Gazette of India.

Supply of Copies of the State Medical Registers

22.

Each State Medical Council shall supply to the Council six printed copies of the State Medical Register as soon as may be after the commencement of this Act and subsequently after the first day of April of each year, and each Registrar of a State Medical Council shall inform the Council without delay of all additions to and other amendments in the State Medical Register made from time to time.

Registration in the Indian Medical Register

23.

The Registrar of the Council, may, on receipt of the report of registration of a person in a State Medical Register or on application made in the prescribed manner by any such person, enter his name in the Indian Medical Register, Provided that the Registrar is satisfied that the person concerned possesses a recognised medical qualification.

Removal of Names from the Indian Medical Register

24.

1. If the name of any person enrolled on a State Medical

Register is removed there from in pursuance of any power conferred by or under any law relating to medical practitioners for the time being in force in any State, the Council shall direct the removal of the name of such person from the Indian Medical Register.

2. Where the name of any person has been removed from a State Medical Register on the ground of professional misconduct or any other ground except that he is not possessed of the requisite medical qualifications or where any application made by the said person for restoration of his name to the State Medical Register has been rejected, he may appeal in the prescribed manner and subject to such conditions including conditions as to the payment of a fee as may be laid down in rules made by the Central Government in this behalf, to the Central Government, whose decision, which shall be given after consulting the Council, shall be binding on the State Government and on the authorities concerned with the preparation of the State Medical Register.

Provisional Registration

25.

1. A citizen of India possessing a medical qualification granted by a medical institution outside India included in part II of the Third Schedule, who is required to undergo practical training as prescribed under sub section (3) of Section 13, shall, on production of proper evidence that he has been selected for such practical training in an approved institution be entitled to be registered provisionally in a State Medical Register and shall be entitled to practice medicine in the approved institution for

the purposes of such training and for no other purpose.

2. A person who has passed the qualifying examination of any university or Medical Institution in India for the grant of a recognized medical qualification shall be entitled to be registered provisionally in a State Medical Register for the purpose of enabling him to be engaged in employment in a resident medical capacity in any approved institution, or in the Medical Service of the Armed Forces of the Union, and for no other purpose, on production of proper evidence that he has been selected for such employment.
3. The names of all persons provisionally registered under sub-section (1) or sub-section (2) in the State Medical Register shall be entered therein separately from the names of other persons registered therein.
4. A person registered provisionally as aforesaid who has completed practical training referred to in sub section (1) or who has been engaged for the prescribed period in employment in a resident medical capacity in any approved institution or in the Medical service of the Armed Forces of the Union, as the case may be, shall be entitled to registration in the State Medical Register under Section 15.

Registration of Additional Qualifications

26.

1. If any person whose name is entered in the Indian Medical Register obtains any title, diploma or other qualification for proficiency in sanitary science, public health or medicine which is a recognized medical qualification, he shall, on application made in this behalf in the prescribed manner be entitled to have

any entry stating such other title, diploma or other qualification made against his name in the Indian Medical Register either in substitution for or in addition to any entry previously made.

2. The entries in respect of any such person in a State Medical Register shall be altered in accordance with the alterations made in the Indian Medical Register.

Privileges of Persons Who are Enrolled on the Indian Medical Register

27.

Subject to the conditions and restrictions laid down in this Act, regarding medical practice by persons possessing certain recognised medical qualifications, every person whose name is for the time being borne on the Indian Medical Register shall be entitled according to his qualifications to practice as a medical practitioner in any part of India and to recover in due course of law in respect of such practice any expenses, charges in respect of medicaments or other appliances, or any fees to which he may be entitled.

Persons Enrolled on the Indian Medical Register to Notify Change of Place of Residence or Practice

28.

Every person registered in the Indian Medical Register shall notify any transfer of the place of his residence or practice to the Council and to the State Medical Council concerned, within thirty days of such transfer failing which his right to participate in the election of members to the Council or a State Medical Council shall be liable to be forfeited by order of the Central Government either permanently or for such period as may be specified therein.

INformation to be Furnished by the Council and Publication Thereof

29.

1. The Council shall furnish such reports, copies of its minutes, abstracts of its accounts, and other information to the Central Government as that Government may require.
2. The Central Government may publish in such manner as it may think fit, any report, copy, abstract or other information furnished to it under this section or under sections 17 and 18.

Commission of Inquiry

30.

1. Whenever it is made to appear to the Central Government that the Council is not complying with any of the provisions of this Act, the Central Government may refer the particulars of the complaint to a Commission of Inquiry consisting of three persons two of whom shall be appointed by the Central Government, one being a Judge of a High Court and one by the Council, and such Commission shall proceed to inquire in a summary manner and to report to the Central Government as to the truth of the matters charged in the complaint, and in case of any charge of default or of improper action being found by the commission to have been established, the Commission shall recommend the remedies, if any, which are in its opinion necessary.
2. The Central Government may require the Council to adopt the remedies so recommended within such time as, having regard to the report of the Commission, it may think fit, and if the Council

fails to comply with any such requirement, the Central Government may amend the regulations of the Council, or make such provision or order or take such other steps as may seem necessary to give effect to the recommendations of the Commission.

3. A Commission of inquiry shall have power to administer oaths, to enforce the attendance of witnesses and the production of documents, and shall have all such other necessary powers for the purpose of any inquiry conducted by it as are exercised by a Civil Court under the Code of Civil Procedure, 1908.

Protection of Action Taken in Good Faith

31.

No suit, prosecution or other legal proceeding shall lie against the Government, the Council or a State Medical Council or any Committee thereof, or any Officer or servant of the Government or Councils aforesaid for anything which is in good faith done or intended to be done under this Act.

Power to Make Rules

32.

1. The Central Government may, by notification in the Official Gazette, make rules to carry out the purposes of this Act.
2. All rules made under this section shall be laid for not less than thirty days before both Houses of Parliament as soon as possible after they are made, and shall be subject to such modifications as Parliament may make during the session in which they are so laid or the session immediately following.

Power to Make Regulations

33. The Council may, with the previous sanction of the Central Government, make regulations generally to carry out the purposes of this Act, and without prejudice to the generality of this power, such regulations may provide for:-

(a) the management of the property of the Council and the maintenance and audit of its accounts;

(b) the summoning and holding of meetings of the Council, the times and places where such meetings are to be held, the conduct of business thereat and the number of members necessary to constitute a quorum;

(c) the resignation of members of the Council;

(d) the powers and duties of the President and Vice-President

(e) the mode of appointment of the Executive Committee and other Committees, the summoning and holding of meetings and the conduct of business of such Committees;

(f) the tenure office, and the powers and duties of the Registrar and other officers and servants of the Council; (fa) the form of the scheme, the particulars to be given in such scheme, the manner in which the scheme is to be preferred and the fee payable with the scheme under clause (b) of sub-section (2) of section 10A; (fb) any other factors under clause (g) of sub-section (7) of section 10A; (fc) the criteria for identifying a student who has been granted a medical qualification referred to in the Explanation to sub-section (3) of section 10B;

(g) the particulars to be stated, and the proof of

qualifications to be given in applications for registration under this Act;

(h) the fees to be paid on applications and appeals under this Act;

(i) the appointment, powers, duties and procedure of medical inspectors and visitors;

(j) the courses and period of study and of practical training to be undertaken, the subjects of examination and the standards of proficiency therein to be obtained, in Universities or medical institutions for grant of recognized medical qualifications;

(k) the standards of staff, equipment, accommodation, training and other facilities for medical education;

(l) the conduct of professional examination; qualifications of examiners and the conditions of admissions to such examinations;

(m) the standards of professional conduct and etiquette and code of ethics to be observed by medical practitioners; and (m a) the modalities for conducting screening tests under sub-section (4A), and under the proviso to sub-section (4B), and for issuing eligibility certificate under sub-section (4B), of section 13,.

(n) any matter for which under this Act provision may be made by regulations.

Repeal of Act 27 of 1933

34.

1. The Indian Medical Council Act, 1933 is hereby repealed.

2. Notwithstanding anything contained in this Act, until the Council is constituted in accordance with the provisions of this Act:-

   (a) the Medical Council of India as constituted immediately before the commencement of this Act under the Indian Medical Council Act, 1933, with the addition of seven members nominated thereto by the Central Government from among persons enrolled on any of the State Medical Registers who possess the medical qualifications included in Part I of the 3rd Schedule to this Act (hereinafter referred to as the said Medical Council) shall be deemed to be the Council constituted under this Act and may exercise any of the powers conferred or perform any of the duties imposed on the Council; and any vacancy occurring in the said Medical Council may be filled up in such manner as Central Govt. may think fit; and

   (b) the Executive Committee and other Committees of the said Medical Council as constituted immediately before the commencement of this Act, shall be deemed to be the Executive Committee and the Committees constituted under this Act.

[Published in the Gazette of India – Part II Section 1 No. 54 Dated April, 3 1993]

MINISTRY OF LAW, JUSTICE AND COMPANY AFFAIRS

(Legislative Department)

New Delhi, the 3rd April, 1993 / Chaitra 13, 1915 (Saka)

The following Act of Parliament received the assent of the President on the 2nd April 1993, and is hereby published for general information:

The Indian Medical Council (Amendment) Act, 1993

No. 31 of 1993 (2nd April, 1993)

An Act further to amend the Indian Medical Council Act, 1956. Be it enacted by Parliament in the Forty fourth year of the Republic of India as follows:- Short title and commencement

1.

(1) The Act may be called the Indian Medical Council (Amendment) Act, 1993.

(2) It shall be deemed to have come into force on the 27th day of August. 1992.

Insertion of new sections 10A, 10B and 10C

2. After section 10 of the Indian Medical Council Act 1956 (hereinafter referred to as the principal Act), [102 of 1956] the following sections shall be inserted namely:-

PERMISSION FOR ESTABLISHMENT OF NEW MEDICAL COLLEGE NEW COURSE OF STUDY ETC.

10A.

(1) Notwithstanding anything contained in this Act or any other law for the time being in force:-

(a) no person shall establish a medical college; or

(b) no medical college shall-

(i) open a new or higher course of study or training (including a post-graduate course of study or training) which would enable a student of such course or training to qualify himself for the award of any recognised medical qualification; or

(ii) increase its admission capacity in any course of study or training (including a post-graduate course of study or training).

except with the previous permission of the Central Government obtained in accordance with the provisions of this section.

Explanation 1 – for the purposes of this section, "person" includes any University or a trust but does not include the Central Government. Explanation 2. – For the purposes of this section. "admission capacity" in relation to any course of study or training (including post-graduate course of study or training) in a medical college, means the maximum number of students that may be fixed by the Council from time to time for being admitted to such course or training.

(2)

(a) Every person or medical college shall, for the purpose of obtaining permission under sub-section (1), submit to the Central Government a scheme in accordance with the provisions of clause (b) and the Central Government shall refer the scheme to the Council for its recommendations.

(b) The scheme referred to in clause (a) shall be in such form and contain such particulars and be [preferred in such manner and be accompanied with such fee as may be prescribed.

(3) On receipt of a scheme by the Council under sub-section (2), the Council may obtain such other particulars as may be considered necessary by it from the person or the medical college concerned and thereafter, it may-

(a) if the scheme is defective and does not contain any necessary particulars give a reasonable opportunity

to the person or college concerned for making a written representation and it shall be open to such person or medical college to rectify the defects, if any, specified by the Council;

(b) consider the scheme having regard to the factors referred to in sub-section (7), and submit the scheme together with its recommendations thereon to the Central Government.

(4) The Central Government may after considering the scheme and the recommendations of the Council under sub-section (3) and after obtaining, where necessary, such other particulars as may be considered necessary by it from the person or college concerned and having regard to the factors referred to in sub-section (1), either approve (with such conditions, if any, as it may consider necessary) or disapprove the scheme and any such approval shall be a permission under sub-section (1) provided that no scheme shall be disapproved by the Central Government except after giving the person or college concerned a reasonable opportunity of being heard: Provided further that nothing in this sub-section shall prevent any person or medical college whose scheme has not been approved by the Central Government to submit a fresh scheme and the provisions of this section shall apply to such scheme as if such scheme has been submitted for the first time under sub-section (2)

(5) Where, within a period of one year from the date of submission of the scheme to the Central Government under sub-section (2), no order passed by the Central Government has been approved by the Central Government in the form in which it has been submitted and accordingly, the permission of the Central Government required under sub-section (1) shall also be deemed to have been granted.

(6) In computing the time-limit specified in sub-section (5), the time taken by the person or college concerned submitting the scheme in furnishing any particulars called for by the Council, or by Central Government, shall be excluded.

(7) The Council, while making its recommendations under clause (b) of sub-section (3) and the Central Government while passing on order, either approving or disapproving the scheme under sub-section (4), shall have due regard to the following factors, namely:-

(a) whether the proposed medical college or the existing medical college seeking to open a now or higher course of study or training, would be in a position, to offer the minimum standards of medical education as prescribed by the Council under section 19A or, as the case may be, under section 20 in the case of post-graduate medical education.

(b) whether the person seeking to establish a medical college or the existing medical college seeking to open a new or higher course of study or training or to increase its admission capacity has adequate financial resources:

(c) whether necessary facilities in respect of staff, equipment, training and other facilities to ensure proper functioning of the medical college or conducting the new course of study or training or accommodating the increased admission capacity have been provided or would be provided within the time-limit specified in the scheme:

(d) whether adequate hospital facilities, having regard to the number of students likely to attend such medical college or course of study or training or as a result of the increased admission capacity, have been provided or would be provided within the time-limit specified in the scheme:

(e) whether any arrangement has been made or programme drawn to impart proper training to students likely to attend such medical college or course of study or training by persons having the recognised medical qualifications;

(f) the requirement of manpower in the field of practice of medicine; and

(g) any other factors as may be prescribed.

(8) Where the Central Government passes an order either approving or disapproving a scheme under this section, a copy of the order shall be communicated to the person or college concerned.

Non-recognition of Medical Qualifications in Certain Cases

10B.

1. Where any medical college is established except with the previous permission of the Central Government in accordance with the provision of section 10A, no medical qualification granted to any student of such medical college shall be a recognised medical qualification for the purposes of this Act.
2. Where any medical college opens a new or higher course of study or training (including a post-graduate course of study or training) except with the previous permission of the Central Government in accordance with the provisions of section 10A, no medical qualification granted to any student of such medical college on the basis of such study or training shall be a recognised medical qualification for the purposes of this Act.

3. Where any medical college increases its admission capacity in any course of study or training except with the previous permission of the Central Government in accordance with the provision of section 10A, no medical qualification granted to any student of such medical college on the basis of the increase in its admission capacity shall be a recognised medical qualification for the purposes of this Act.

Explanation – For the purposes of this section, the criteria for identifying a student who has been granted a medical qualification on the basis of such increase in the admission capacity shall be such as may be prescribed.

Time for seeking permission for certain existing medical colleges etc.

10C.

1. If, after the 1st day of June, 1992 and on and before the commencement of the Indian Medical Council (Amendment) Act, 1993 any person has established a medical college or any medical college has opened a new or higher course of study or training or increased the admission capacity, such person or medical college, as the case may be, shall seek, within a period of one year from the commencement of the Indian Medical Council (Amendment) Act, 1993, the permission of the Central Government in accordance with the provisions of section 10A.

If any person or medical college, as the case may be fails to seek the permission under sub-section (1), the provisions of section 10B shall apply, so far as may be as if, permission of the Central Government under section 10A has been refused.

2.

Amendment of Section 33

3. In section 32 of the principal Act, after clause (f) the following clauses shall be inserted, namely:-

"(fa) the form of the scheme, the particulars to be given in such scheme, the manner in which the scheme is to be preferred and the fee payable with the scheme under clause (b) of sub-section (2) of section 10A;

(fb) any other factors under clause (g) of sub-section (7) of section 10A;

(fc) the criteria for identifying a student who has been granted a medical qualification referred to in the Explanation to sub-section (3) of section 10B".

Repeal and Saving

4.

(1) The Indian Medical Council (Amendment) Ordinance, 1993 (ORD 2 of 1993) is hereby repealed. (2) Notwithstanding such repeal, anything done or any action taken under the principal Act, as amended by the said Ordinance, shall be deemed to have been done or taken under the principal Act, as amended by this Act.

B.R. ATRE
Joint Secy. to the Govt. of India.

THE GAZETTE OF INDIA EXTRAORDINARY

Published by Authority

No. 41 New Delhi: Monday, September 3, 2001/BHADRA 12, 1923

Ministry of Law, Justice and Company Affairs (Legislative Department)

New Delhi, the 3rd September, 2001/Bhadra 12, 1923 (Saka)

The following Act of Parliament received the assent of the President on the 3rd September, 2001, and is hereby published for general information:-

The Indian Medical Council (Amendment) Act, 2001

(Act No. 34 of 2001)

[3rd September, 2001]

An Act further to amend the Indian Medical Council Act, 1956. Be it enacted by Parliament in the Fifty-second Year of the Republic of India as follows: Short Title

This Act may be called the India Medical Council (Amendment) Act, 2001.

Amendment of Section 13

2. In the Indian Medical Council Act, 1956 (102 of 1956) (hereinafter referred to as the principal Act, in section 13, -
   (a) in sub-section (3), after the words "granted by medical institutions outside India", the words "before such date as the Central Government may, by notification in the Official Gazette, specify" shall be inserted;
   (b) in sub-section (4), the following provisos and Explanation shall be inserted at the end, namely:-

Provided that after the commencement of the Indian Medical Council (Amendment) Act, 2001, no such amendment shall be made in Part II of the Third Schedule to include any primary medical qualification granted by any medical institution outside India:

Provided further that nothing contained in the first proviso shall apply to inclusion in Part II of the Third Schedule any primary medical qualification granted by any medical institution outside India to any person whose name is entered in the Indian Medical Register.

Explanation- For the purposes of this sub-section, "primary medical qualification" means any minimum qualification sufficient for enrolment on any State Medical Register or for entering the name in the Indian Medical Register.

(4A) A person who is a citizen of India and obtains medical qualification granted by any medical institution in any country outside India recognised for enrolment as medical practitioner in that country after such date as may be specified by the Central GovMedical Register maintained by a State Medical Council or to have his name entered in the Indian Medical Register unless he qualified the screening test in India prescribed for such purpose and such foreign medical qualification after such person qualifies that said screening test shall be deemed to be the recognised medical qualification for the purposes of this Act for that person.

(4B) A person who is a citizen of India shall not, after such date as may be specified by the Central Government under sub-section (3), be eligible to get admission to obtain medical qualification granted by any medical institution in any foreign country without obtaining an eligibility certificate issued to him by the Council and in case any such person obtains such qualification without obtaining such eligibility certificate, he shall not be eligible to appear in the screening test referred to in sub-section (4A):

Provided that an Indian citizen who has acquired the medical qualification from foreign medical institution or has obtained admission in foreign medical institution before the commencement of the Indian Medical Council (Amendment) Act, 2001 shall not be required to obtain eligibility certificate under this sub-section but, if he is qualified for admission to any medical course for recognised medical qualification in any medical institution in India, he shall be required to qualify only the screening test prescribed for enrolment on any State Medical Register or for entering his name in the Indian Medical Register.

(4C) Nothing contained in sub-sections (4A) and (4B) shall apply to the medical qualifications referred to in section 14 for the purposes of that section.

Amendment of Section 33

1. In section 33 of the principal Act, after clause (m), the following clause shall be inserted, namely:-

> "(ma) the modalities for conducting screening tests under the sub-section (4A), and under the proviso to sub-section (4B), and for issuing eligibility certificate under sub-section (4B), of section 13,".

Subhash C. Jain
Secy. to the Govt. of India

THE INDIAN MEDICINE CENTRAL COUNCIL ACT, 1970

(Act No. 48 of 1970) 21st December, 1970.

An Act to provide for the constitution of a Central Council of Indian Medicine and the maintenance of a Central Register of Indian Medicine and for matter connected therewith.

Be it enacted by Parliament in the twenty-first year of the Republic of India as follows:-

I. PRELIMINARY

(1) Short Title, Extent and Commencement

(1) This Act may be called the Indian Medicine Central Council Act, 1970.

(2) It extends to the whole of India.

(3) It shall come into force in a State on such date as the Central Govt. may be notification in the Official Gazette, appoint in this behalf for such State, and different dates may be appointed for different States and for different provision of this Act.

(2) Definition -

(1) In this Act, unless the context otherwise requires,

(a) "approve institution" means a teaching institution, health center or hospital recognized by a University or board as an institution in which a person may undergo the training, if any, required by his course of study before the award of any medical qualification to him;

(b) "Board" means a Board, Council, Examining Body or Faculty of Indian Medicine (by whatever name called) constituted by the State Govt. under any law for the time being in force regulating the award of medical qualifications in, and registration of practitioners of, Indian medicine;

(c) "Central Council" means the Central Council of Indian Medicine constituted under section 3;

(d) "Central Register of India Medicine, means the register maintained by the Central Council under this Act.

(e) "Indian Medicine" means the system of Indian medicine commonly known as Ashtang Ayurveda, Siddha or Unani Tibb whether supplemented or not by such modern advances as the Central Council may declare by notification from time to time.

(f) "Medical institution" means any institution within or without India, which grants degrees, diploma or license in Indian medicine.

(g) "prescribed" means prescribed by regulation;

(h) "recognized medical qualification' means any of the medical qualifications, including Post-Graduate medical qualification, of Indian medicine included in the Second, Third or Fourth Schedule;

(i) "regulation" means a regulation made under section 36;

(j) "State Register of Indian Medicine" means a register or registers maintained under any law for the time being in force in any State regulating the registration of practitioners of Indian Medicine;

(k) "University" means any university in India established by law and having a Faculty of Indian Medicine and includes a University in India established by law in which instruction, teaching, training or research in Indian medicine is provided.

(2) Any reference in this Act to a law which is not in force in the State of Jammu and Kashmir shall, in relation to that State, be construed as a reference to the corresponding law, if any, in force in that State.

II. THE CENTRAL COUNCIL AND ITS COMMITTEES

(3) Constitution of Central Council

(1) The Central Govt. shall, by notification in the Official

Gazette constitute for the purposes of this act a Central Council Consisting of the following members, namely:-

(a) such number of members not exceeding five as may be determined by the Central Govt. in accordance with the provisions of the First Schedule for each of the Ayurveda, Siddha and Unani systems of medicine from each State in which a State Register of Indian Medicine is maintained, to be elected from amongst themselves by persons enrolled on that Register as practitioners of Ayurveda, Siddha or Unani, as the case may be;

(b) one member for each of the Ayurveda, Siddha and Unani systems of medicine from each University to be elected from amongst themselves by the members of the Faculty or Department (by whatever name called) of the respective system of medicine of that University;

(c) such number of members, not exceeding thirty percent of the total number of members elected under clauses(a) and (b), as may nominated by the Central Govt., from amongst persons having special knowledge or practical experience in respect of Indian medicine;

Provided that until member are elected under clause (a) or clause (b) in accordance with the provision of this Act and the rules made thereunder, the Central Govt. shall nominate such number of member, being persons qualified to be chosed as such under the said clause (a) or clause (b), as the case may be, as that Govt. thinks fit; and references to elected members in this Act shall be construed as including references to members so nominated.

(2) The President of the Central Council shall be elected by the members of the Central Council from amongst

themselves in such manner as may be prescribed.

(3) There shall be a Vice-President for each of the Ayurveda, Siddha and Unani system of medicine who shall be elected from amongst themselves by members representing that system of medicine, elected under clause (a) or clause (b) of sub-section (1) or nominated under clause (c) of that sub-section.

(4) Mode of Election

(1) An election under clause (a) or clause (b) of sub-section (1) of section 3 shall be conducted by the Central Govt. in accordance with such rules as may be made by it in this behalf.

(2) Where any dispute arises regarding any election to the Central Council, it shall be referred to the Central Govt. whose decision shall be final.

(5) Restriction of Elections and Membership

(1) No person shall be eligible for election to the Central Council unless he possesses any of the medical qualification included in the Second, Third or Fourth Schedule, is enrolled on any State Register of Indian Medicine and resides in the State concerned.

(2) No person may at the same time serve as a member in more than one capacity.

(6) Incorporation of Central Council

The Central Council shall be a body corporate by the name of Central Council of Indian Medicine having perpetual succession and a common seal, with power to acquire, hold and dispose of property, both movable and immovable and to contract, and shall by the said name sue and be sued.

(7) Term of Office of President, Vice-President and Members of Central Council

(1) The President, a Vice-President or a member of the Central Council shall hold office for a term of five years from the date of his election or nomination, as the case may be, or until his successor shall have been duly elected or nominated, whichever is longer.

(2) An elected or nominated member shall be deemed to have vacated his seat if he is absent without excuse, sufficient in the opinion of the Central Council, from three consecutive ordinary meeting of the Central Council or, in the case of a member elected under clause (a) of sub-section (1) of Section 3, if he ceases to be enrolled on the concerned State Register of Indian Medicine, or in the case of a member elected under clause (b) of that sub-section, if he ceases to be member of faculty or Department (by whatever name called) of Indian medicine of the University concerned.

(3) A casual vacancy in the Central Council shall be filled by election or nomination, as the case may be, and the person elected or nominated to fill the vacancy shall hold office only for the remainder of the term for which the member whose place he takes was elected or nomination.

(4) Member of the Central Council shall be eligible for re-election or re-nomination.

(5) Where the said term of five year is about to expire in respect of any member, a successor may be elected or nominated at any time within three months before the said term expires but he shall not assume office until the said term has expired.

(8) Meeting of Central Council

(1) The Central Council shall meet at least once in each

year at such time and place as may be appointed by the Central Council.

(2) Unless otherwise prescribed, one-third of the total number of members of the Central Council shall form a quorum and all the acts of the Central Council shall be decided by a majority of the members present and voting:-

> Provided that no decision of the Central Council in relation to any Indian medicine, shall be effective unless three members representing Ayurveda, Siddha or Unani system of medicine as the case may be, are present at the meeting and support the decision.

(9) Committees for Ayurveda, Siddha and Unani

(1) The Central Council shall constitute from amongst its members:-

(a) a committee for Ayurveda

(b) a committee for Siddha and

(c) a committee for Unani,

and each such committee shall consist of members elected under clause(a) or clause(b) or nominated under clause (c) of sub-section (1) of section 3 representing the Ayurveda, Siddha or Unani System of medicine, as the case may be.

(2) The Vice-President for each of the Ayurveda, Siddha and Unani System of medicine elected under sub-section (3) of section 3 shall be, respectively, the Chairman of the committees referred to in clauses (a), (b) and (c) of sub-section (1).

(3) Subject to each general or special directions as the Central Council may from time to time give, each such committee shall be competent to deal with any matter

relating to Ayurveda, Siddha or Unani system of medicine, as the case may be, within the competence of the Central Council.

(10) Other Committees

The Central Council may constitute from amongst its members such other committees for general or special purposes, as the Central Council deems necessary to carry out the purposes of this Act.

(11) Meetings of Committees

(1) The committees constituted under section 9 and 10 shall meet at least once in each year at such time and place as may be appointed by the Central Council.

(2) Unless otherwise prescribed, one-third of the total number of members of a committee shall form a quorum, and all the acts of the committee shall be decided by a majority of the members present and voting.

(12) Officers and Other Employees of Central Council

The Central Council shall:-

(a) appoint a Registrar who shall act as Secretary and who may also, if deemed expedient, act as Treasure.

(b) employ such other persons as it deems necessary to carry out the purposes of this Act;

(c) require and take from the Registrar, or from any employee, such security for the due performance of his duties as the Central Council deems necessary; and

(d) with the previous sanction of the Central Government, fix the remuneration and allowances to be paid to the President, Vice-President and members of the Central Council and to the Members of the committees thereof and determine the conditions of service of the employees of the Central Council.

(13) Vacancies in the Central Council and Committees Thereof Not to Invalidate Acts, etc.

No act or proceeding of the Central Council or any committee thereof shall be called in question on the ground merely of the existence of any vacancy in, or any defect in the constitution of, the Central Council or the committee, as the case may be.

III. RECOGNITION OF MEDICAL QUALIFICATION

(14) Recognition of Medical Qualifications Granted by Certain Medical Institutions in India

(1) The medical qualifications granted by any University, Board or other medical institutions in India which are included in the Second Schedule shall be recognized medical qualifications for the purposes of this Act.

(2) Any University, Board or other medical institution in India which grants a medical qualification not included in the Second Schedule may apply to the Central Govt. to have any such qualification recognized and the Central Govt., after consulting the Central Council, may, be notification in the Official Gazette, amend the Second Schedule so as to include such qualification therein and any such notification may also direct that an entry shall be made in the last column of the Second Schedule against such medical qualification declaring that if shall be recognized medical qualification only when granted after a specified date.

(15) Recognition of Medical Qualifications Granted by Certain Medical Institutions Whose Qualifications are Not Included in Second Schedule

The medical qualifications included in the Third Schedule granted to a citizen of India before the 15th day of August, 1947, by any medical institution in any area which was comprised before that date within India as defined in the Govt. of India Act, 1935, shall also be recognized medical qualification for the purposes of this Act.

(16) Recognition of Medical Qualifications Granted by Medical Institutions in Counties with Which There is a Scheme of Reciprocity

(1) The medical qualifications granted by medical institutions outside India which are included in the Fourth Schedule shall be recognized medical qualifications for the purposes of this Act.

(2)The Central Council may enter into negotiations with the authority in any State or country outside India, which, by law of such State or country is entrusted with the maintenance of a Register of Practitioners of Indian medicine, for the settling of a scheme of reciprocity for the recognition of medical qualifications in Indian medicine and in pursuance of any such scheme, the Central Govt. may, by notification in the Official Gazette, amend the Fourth Schedule so as to include therein any medical qualification which the Central Council has decided should be recognized and any such notification may also direct that an entry shall be made in the last column of the Fourth Schedule against such medical qualification declaring that it shall be recognized medical qualification only when granted after a specified date.

17. Rights of Persons Possessing Qualifications Included in Second, Third and Fourth Schedules to be Enrolled

(1) Subject to the other provisions contained in this Act, any medical qualification included in the Second, Third or Fourth Schedule shall be sufficient qualification for enrolment on any State Register of India Medicine.

(2) Save as provided in section 28, no person other than a practitioner of Indian medicine who possesses a recognized

medical qualification and is enrolled on a State Register or the Central Register of Indian Medicine;-

(a) shall hold office as Vaid, Siddha, Hakim or Physician or any other office (by whatever designation called) in Govt. or in any institution maintained by a local or other authority;

(b) shall practice Indian medicine in any State;

(c) shall be entitled to sign or authenticate a medical or fitness certificate or any other certificate required by any law to be signed or authenticated by a duly qualified medical practitioner;

(d) shall be entitled to give evidence at any inquest or in any court of law as an expert under section 45 of the Indian Evidence Act, 1872 (1 of 1872) on any matter relating to Indian medicine.

(3) Nothing contained in sub-section (2) shall affect;-

(a) The right of a practitioner of Indian Medicine enrolled on a State Register of Indian Medicine to practice Indian medicine in any State merely on the ground that, on the commencement of this Act, he does not possess a recognized medical qualification.

(b) The privileges (including the right to practice any system of medicine) conferred by or under any law relating to registration of practitioners of Indian medicine for the time being in force in any State on a practitioner of Indian Medicine enrolled on a State Register of Indian medicine;

(c) The right of a person to practice Indian medicine in a State in which, on the commencement of this Act, a State Register of Indian Medicine is not maintained if, on such commencement, he has been practicing Indian medicine for not less than five years

(d) The rights conferred by or under the Indian Medical Council Act, 1956 (102 of 1956) [including the right to practice medicine as defined in clause (f) of section 2 of the said Act], on persons possessing any qualifications included in the Schedules to the said Act.

(4) Any person who acts in contravention of any provision of sub-section (2) shall be punished with imprisonment for a term which may extend to one year, or with fine which may extend to one thousand rupees, or with both.

(18) Power to Require Information as to Courses of Study and Examination

Every University, Board or medical institution in India which grants a recognized medical qualification shall furnish such information as the Central Council may, from time to time, require as to the courses of study and examinations to be undergone in order to obtain such qualification, as to the ages at which such courses of study and examinations are required to be undergone and such qualification is conferred and generally as to the requisites for obtaining such qualification.

(19) Inspectors at Examinations

(1) The Central Council shall appoint such number of medical inspectors as it may deem requisite to inspect any medical college, hospital or other institutions where education in India medicine is given, or to attend any examination held by any University, Board or medical institution for the purpose of recommending to the Central Govt. recognition of medical qualifications granted by that University, Board or medical institute.

(2) The medical inspectors shall not interfere with the conduct of any training of examination, but shall report to

the Central Council on the adequacy of the standards of education including staff, equipment, accommodation, training and other facilities prescribed for giving education in Indian medicine or on the sufficiency of every examination which they attend.

(3) The Central Council shall forward a copy of any such report to the University, Board or medical institution concerned and shall also forward a copy with the remarks of the University, Board or medical institution thereon, to the Central Govt.

(20) Visitors at Examinations

(1) The Central Council may appoint such number of visitors as it may deem requisite to inspect any medical college, hospital or other institution where education in Indian medicine is given or to attend any examination for the purpose of granting recognized medical qualifications.

(2) Any person, whether he a member of the Central Council or not, may be appointed as a visitor under this section but a person who is appointed as an inspector under Section 19 for any inspection or examination shall not be appoint as a visitor for the same inspection or examination.

(3) The visitors shall not interfere with the conduct of any training or examination, but shall report to the President of the Central Council on the adequacy of the standards of education including staff, equipment, accommodation, training and other facilities prescribed for giving education in Indian medicine or on the sufficiency of every examination which they attend.

(4) The report of a visitor shall be treated as confidential unless in any particular case the President of Central Council otherwise directs:-

Provided that if the Central Govt. requires a copy of the report of a visitor, the Central Council shall furnish the same.

21. Withdrawal of Recognition

(1) When upon report by the inspector or the visitor, it appears to the Central Council;-

(a) that the courses of study and examination to be undergone in, or the proficiency required from candidates at any examination held by, any University, Board or medical institution, or

(b) that the staff, equipment, accommodation, training and other facilities for instruction and training provided in such University, Board or medical institution or in any college or other institution affiliated to the University.

Do not conform to the standard prescribed by the Central Council the Central Council shall make a representation to that effect to the Central Govt.

(2) After considering such representation, the Central Govt. may send it to the Govt. of the State in which the University, Board or medical institution is situated and the State Govt. shall forward it along, with such remarks as it may choose to make to the University, Board or medical institution, with an intimation of the period within which the University, Board or medical institution may submit its explanation to the State Govt.

(3) On the receipt of the explanation or, where no explanation is submitted within the period fixed, then, on the expiry of that period, the State Govt. shall make its recommendations to the Central Govt.

(4) The Central Govt., after making such further inquiry,

if any, as it may think fit, may, by notification in the Official Gazette, direct that an entry shall be made in the appropriate Schedule against the said medical qualification declaring that it shall be a recognized medical qualification only when granted before a specified date, or that the said medical qualification if granted to students of a specified college or institution affiliated to any University shall be recognized medical qualification only when granted before a specified date or, as the case may be, that the said medical qualification shall be recognized medical qualification in relation to a specified college or institution affiliated to any University only when granted after a specified date.

(22) Minimum Standards of Education in Indian Medicine

(1) The Central Council may prescribe the minimum standards of education in Indian medicine, required for granting recognized medical qualifications by Universities, Boards or medical institutions in India.

(2) Copies of the draft regulation and of all subsequent amendments thereof shall be furnished by the Central Council to all State Government and the Central Council shall, before submitting the regulation or any amendment thereof, as the case may be, to the Central Govt. for sanction, take into consideration the comments of any State Govt. received within three months from the furnishing of the copies as aforesaid.

(3) Each of the committees referred to in clauses (a),(b) and (c) of sub-section (1) of Section 9 shall, from time to time, report to the Central Council on the efficacy of the regulations and may recommend to the Central Council such amendments thereof as it may think it.

IV. THE CENTRAL REGISTER OF INDIAN MEDICINE

(23) The Central Register of Indian Medicine

(1) The Central Council shall cause to maintained in the prescribed manner, a register of practitioners in separate part for each of the system of Indian medicine to be known as the Central Register of Indian medicine which shall contain the names of all persons who are for the time being enrolled on any State Register of Indian Medicine and who possess any of the recognized medical qualifications.

(2) It shall be the duty of the Registrar of the Central Council to keep and maintain the Central Register of Indian Medicine in accordance with the provisions of this Act and of any orders made by the Central Council and from time to time to revise the register and publish it in the Gazette of Indian in such other manner as may be prescribed.

(3) Such register shall be deemed to be a public document within the meaning of the Indian Evidence Act, 1872 (1 of 1872) and may be proved by a copy published in the Gazette of India.

(24) Supply of copies of State Register of Indian Medicine

Each Board shall supply to the Central Council three printed copies of the State Register of Indian Medicine as soon as may be after the commencement of this Act and subsequently after the first day of April of each year and each Board shall inform the Central Council without delay of all additions to and other amendments in the State Register of Indian medicine made from time to time:-

(25) Registration in Central Register of Indian Medicine

The Register of the Central Council may on receipt of the report of registration of a person in a State Register of Indian Medicine or on application made in the prescribed manner by any person, enter his name in the Central Register of Indian Medicine, provided that the Register is satisfied that the person concerned is eligible under this Act for such registration.

(26) Professional Conduct

(1) The Central Council may prescribe standards of professional conduct and etiquette and a code of ethics for practitioners of Indian medicine.

(2) Regulations made by the Central Council under sub-section (1) may specify which violations thereof shall constitute infamous conduct in any professional respect, that is to say, professional misconduct and such provision shall have effect not with standing anything contained in any law for the time being in force.

(27) Removal of Names from the Central Register of Indian Medicine

(1) If the name of any person enrolled on a State Register of Indian Medicine is removed there from in pursuance of any power conferred by or under any law relating to registration of practitioners of Indian medicine for the time being in force in any State, the Central Council shall direct the removal of the name of such person from the Central Register of Indian Medicine.

(2) Where the name of any person has been removed from a State Register of Indian Medicine on any ground other than that he is not possessed of the requisite medical qualifications or where any application by the said person for restoration of his name to the State Register of Indian Medicine has been rejected, he may appeal in the prescribed manner and subject to such conditions, including conditions as to the payment of a fee, as may be prescribed, to the Central Govt. whose decision, which shall be given after

consulting the Central Council, shall be blinding on the State Govt. and on the authorities concerned with the preparation of the State Register of Indian Medicine.

(28) Provisional Registration for Practice

If the course of study to be undergone for obtaining a recognized medical qualification in Indian Medicine include a period of training after a person has passed the qualifying examination and before such qualification is conferred on him, any such person shall, on application made by him in this behalf, be granted provisional registration in a State Register of Unani medicine by Board concerned in order to enable him to practice Indian Medicine in an approved institution for the purpose of such training and for no other purpose for the period aforesaid.

(29) Privileges of Persons Who are Enrolled on the Central Register of Indian Medicine

Subject to the conditions and restrictions laid down in this Act regarding practice of Indian medicine by persons possessing certain recognized medical qualifications, every person whose name is for the time being borne on the Central Register of Indian medicine shall be entitled according to his qualification to practice Indian medicine in any part of India and to recover in due course of law in respect of such practice any expenses, charges in respect of medicaments or other appliances or any fees to which he may be entitled.

(30) Registration of Additional Qualifications

(1) If any person whose name is entered in the Central Register of Indian medicine obtains any title, diploma or other qualifications for proficiency in Indian medicine which is a recognized medical qualification, he shall, on application made in this behalf in the prescribed manner, be entitled to have an entry stating such other title, diploma or other qualification made against his name in the Central Register

of Indian Medicine either in substitution for or in addition to any entry previously made.

(2) The entries in respect of any such person in a State Register of Indian Medicine shall be altered in accordance with the alterations made in the Central Register of Indian Medicine.

(31) Persons Enrolled on Central Register of Indian Medicine to Notify Change of Place of Residence and Practice

Every person registered in the Central Register of Indian Medicine shall notify any transfer of the place of his residence or practice to the Central Council and to the Board concerned, within ninety days of such transfer, failing which his right to participate in the election of members to the Central Council or a Board shall be liable to be forfeited by order of the Central Govt. either permanently or for such period as may be specified therein.

V. MISCELLANEOUS

(32) Information to be Furnished by Central Council and Publication Thereof

(1) The Central Council shall furnish such reports, copies of its minutes, abstracts of its accounts and other information to the Central Govt. as that Govt. may require.

(2) The Central Govt. may publish in such manner, as it may think fit, any report, copy, abstract or other information furnished to it under this section or under section 20.

(33) Commission of Inquiry

(1) Whenever it is made to appear to the Central Govt. that the Central Council is not complying with any of the provisions of this Act, the Central Govt. may refer the particulars of the complaint to a commission of inquiry consisting of three persons, two of whom shall be appointed

by the Central Govt., one being a judge of a High Court and one by the Central Council and such commission shall proceed to inquire in a summary manner to report to the Central Govt. as to the truth of the matters charged in the complaint and in case of any charge of default or of improper action being found by the commission to have been established, the commission shall recommend the remedies, it any, which are in its opinion necessary.

(2) The Central Govt. may require the Central Govt. to adopt the remedies so recommended within such time as, having regards to the report of the commission, it may think fit and if the Central Council fails to comply with any such requirement, the Central Govt. may amend the regulations of the Central Council, or make such provision or order or take such other steps as may seem necessary to give effect to the recommendations of the commission.

(3) A commission of inquiry shall have power to administer oaths, to enforce the attendance of witnesses and the production of documents and shall have all such other necessary powers for the purpose of any inquiry conducted by it as are exercised by a civil court under the code of Civil Procedure, 1908 (5 of 1908).

(34) Protection of Action Taken in Good Faith

No suit, prosecution or other legal proceeding shall lie against the Govt., the Central Council or a Board or any committee thereof or any officer or servant of the Govt. or the Central Council or the Board aforesaid for anything which is in good faith done or intended to be done under this Act.

(35) Power to Make Rules

(1) The Central Govt. may be notification in the Official Gazette, make rules to carry out the purposes of this Act.

(2) Every rule made under this section shall be laid, as soon as may be after it is made, before each House of Parliament while it is in session for a total period of thirty days which may be comprised in one session or [in tow or more successive sessions and if, before the expiry of the session immediately following the session or the successive sessions aforesaid] both Houses agree in making any modification in the rule or both Houses agree that the rule should not be made the rule shall thereafter have effect only in such modified form or be of no effect, as the case may be; so however, that any such modification or annulment shall be without prejudice to the validity of anything previously done under that rule.

(36) Power to Make Regulations

(1) The Central Council, may, with the previous sanction of the Central Govt., [by notification in the Official Gazette] make regulations generally to carry out the purposes of this Act and without prejudice to the generally of this power, such regulations may provide for-

- (a) the manner of election of the President and the Vice-Presidents of the Central Council;
- (b) the management of the property of the Central Council and the maintenance and audit of its accounts;
- (c) the resignation members of the Central Council;
- (d) the powers and duties of the President and Vice-President;
- (e) the summoning and holding of meetings of the Central Council and the committees thereof, the times and places, where such meetings are to be held and the conduct of business threat and the number of members necessary to constitute a quorum;

(f) the functions of the committees constituted under section 9 or section 10;

(g) the tenure of office and the powers and duties of the Registrar and other officers and servants of the Central Council;

(h) the appointment, powers, duties and procedure of inspectors and visitors;

(i) the courses and period of study and of practical training to be undertaken, the subject of examination and the standards of proficiency therein to be obtained, in any university, board or medical institutions for grant of recognized medical qualifications;

(j) the standards of staff, equipment, accommodation, training and other facilities for education in Indian Medicine;

(k) the conduct of professional examination, qualifications of examiners and the conditions of admissions to such examinations;

(l) the standards of professional conduct and etiquette and code of ethics to be observed by practitioners of Indian Medicine;

(m) the particulars to be stated and the proof of qualifications to be given in applications for registration under this Act;

(n) the manner in which and the conditions subject to which an appeal under section 27 may be preferred;

(o) The fees to be paid on applications and appeals under this Act; and

(p) any matter for which under this Act provision may be made by regulations;

(2) The Central Govt. shall cause every regulation made under this Act to be laid, as soon as may be after it is made, before each House of Parliament, while it is in session, for a total period of thirty days which may be comprised in one session or in two or more successive sessions and if, before the expiry of the session immediately following the session or the successive sessions aforesaid, both Houses agree in making any modification in the regulation or both Houses agree that the regulation should not be made, the regulation shall thereafter have effect only in such modified form or be of no effect, as the case may be; so, however, that any such modification or annulment shall be without prejudice to the validity of anything previously done under that regulation.

MEDICAL COUNCIL OF INDIA

SALIENT FEATURES OF POSTGRADUATE MEDICAL EDUCATION REGULATIONS, 2000

1. Short Title and Commencement

(i) These regulations may be called "The Postgraduate Medical Education Regulations 2000.

(ii) They shall come into force on the date of their publication in the official Gazette.

2. General Conditions to be Observed by Postgraduate Teaching Institutions

(iii) Postgraduate Medical Education in broad specialities shall be of three years duration in the case of degree course and two years in the case of Diploma course after MBBS and in the case of super specialities the duration shall be of three years after MD/MS with the exceptions wherever indicated.

(iv) Postgraduate curriculum shall be competency based.

(v) Learning in postgraduate programme shall be essentially autonomous and self directed.

(vi) A combination of both formative and summative assessment is vital for the successful completion of the PG programme.

(vii) A modular approach to the course curriculum is essential for achieving a systematic exposure to the various sub-specialities concerned with a discipline.

(viii) The training of PG students shall involve learning experience 'derived from' or 'targeted to' the needs of the community. It shall, therefore, be necessary to expose the students to community based activities.

3. Goals And General Objectives of Postgraduate Medical Education Programme to be Observed by Postgraduate Teaching Institution

3.1 Goal

The goal of postgraduate medical education shall be to produce competent specialists and/or Medical teachers.

(i) who shall recognize the health needs of the community, and carry out professional obligations ethically and in keeping with the objectives of the national health policy

(ii) who shall have mastered most of the competencies, pertaining to the speciality, that are required to be practiced at the secondary and the tertiary levels of the health care delivery system;

(iii) who shall be aware of the contemporary advance and developments in the discipline concerned;

(iv) who shall have acquired a spirit of scientific inquiry and is oriented to the principles of research methodology and epidemiology; and

(v) who shall have acquired the basic skills in teaching of the medical and paramedical professionals;

3.2 General Objectives of Post-graduate Training Expected from Students at the End of Post-graduate Training

At the end of the postgraduate training in the discipline concerned the student shall be able to;

(i) Recognize the importance to the concerned speciality in the context of the health needs of the community and the national priorities in the health section.

(ii) Practice the speciality concerned ethically and in step with the principles of primary health care.

(iii) Demonstrate sufficient understanding of the basic sciences relevant to the concerned speciality.

(iv) Identify social, economic, environmental, biological and emotional determinants of health in a given case, and take them into account while planning therapeutic, rehabilitative, preventive and primitive measure/strategies.

(v) Diagnose and manage majority of the conditions in the speciality concerned on the basis of clinical assessment, and appropriately selected and conducted investigations.

(vi) Plan and advise measures for the prevention and rehabilitation of patients suffering from disease and disability related to the speciality.

(vii) Demonstrate skills in documentation of individual case details as well as morbidity and mortality rate relevant to the assigned situation.

(viii) Demonstrate empathy and humane approach towards patients and their families and exhibit interpersonal behaviour in accordance with the societal norms and expectations.

(ix) Play the assigned role in the implementation of national health programme, effectively and responsibly.

(x) Organize and supervise the chosen/assigned health care services demonstrating adequate managerial skills in the clinic/hospital or the field situation.

(xi) Develop skills as a self-directed learner, recognize continuing education needs; select and use appropriate learning resources.

(xii) Demonstrate competence in basic concepts of research methodology and epidemiology, and be able to critically analyze relevant published research literature.

(xiii) Develop skills in using educational methods and techniques as applicable to the teaching of medical/nursing students, general physicians and paramedical health workers.

(xiv) Function as an effective leader of a health team engaged in health care, research or training.

4. Statement of the Competencies

Keeping in view the general objectives of postgraduate training, each discipline shall aim at development of specific competencies which shall be defined and spelt out in clear terms. Each department shall produce a statement and bring it to the notice of the trainees in the beginning of the programme so that he or she can direct the efforts towards the attainment of these competencies.

5. Components of the Postgraduate Curriculum

The major components of the Postgraduate curriculum shall be:

— Theoretical knowledge
— Practical and clinical skills
— Thesis skills.
— Attitudes including communication skills.
— Training in research methodology.

6. Starting of Postgraduate Medical Courses and Their Recognition

(1) An institution intending to start a Postgraduate Medical Education course or to increase the admission capacity shall obtain permission of the Central Government under Section 10A of the Act.

(2) The institution shall apply for recognition of the Postgraduate medical qualification to the Central Government through the affiliating university.

7. Nomenclature of Postgraduate Courses

The nomenclature of postgraduate medical courses shall be as provided in the Schedule annexed to these Regulation:

> Provided that in the case of postgraduate medical degree and diploma courses instituted prior to the commencement of these Regulations with the approval of the Medical Council of India and which have not been included in these regulations, the institutions concerned shall continue such course till the students admitted complete the said courses.

8. General

(1) The institutions recognised by the Medical Council of India for running Postgraduate courses prior to the commencement of the Indian Medical Council (Amendment) Act,1993 and those medical colleges recognised for running Bachelor of Medicine and Bachelor of Surgery (MBBS) course or institutions established by the Central Government for the purpose of imparting postgraduate medical education shall be eligible for starting any postgraduate degree or diploma and higher specialty course.

(1A) The Central Government shall exempt any such existing/proposed non-teaching institutions or specialist institution or autonomous body owned and managed by the

Central Government/State Government from fulfilling the prescribed provision of having an undergraduate teaching facility, and allow starting Postgraduate medical course.

(2) The maximum number of students for a postgraduate medical course, who can be registered in any recognised department, for training for the award of postgraduate degree or diploma by the affiliating university, shall be determined by the facilities available in the department in terms of infrastructure, teaching staff and clinical teaching material.

(3) Every student, selected for admission to postgraduate medical course in any of the medical institutions in the country, shall possess recognised MBBS degree or equivalent qualification and should have obtained permanent Registration with the Medical Council of India, or any of the State Medical Councils or should obtain the same within on month from the date of his admission, failing which the admission of the candidate shall be cancelled;

> Provided that in the case of a foreign national, the Medical Council of India may, on payment of the prescribed fee for registration, grant temporary Registration for the duration of the postgraduate training restricted to the medical college/institution to which he is admitted for the time being exclusively for postgraduate studies; Provided further that temporary registration to such foreign national shall be subject to the condition 5that such person is duly registered as medical practitioner in his own country from which he has obtained his basic medical qualification and that his degree is recognised by the corresponding Medical Council or concerned authority.

(4) The students undergoing postgraduate courses shall be exposed to the following :-

(a) Basics of statistics to understand and critically evaluate published research paper.

(b) Few lectures or other type of exposure to human behavior studies.

(c) Basic understanding of pharmaco-economics.

(d) Introduction to the non-linear mathematics.

9. Selection of Postgraduate Students

(1) Students for Postgraduate medical courses shall be selected strictly on the basis of their academic merit.

(2) For determining the academic merit, the university/ institution may adopt any one of the following procedures both for degree and diploma courses :-

(i) On the basis of merit as determined by the competitive test conducted by the State Government or by the competent authority appointed by the State Government or by the university/group of universities in the same state; or

(ii) On the basis of merit as determined by a centralized competitive test held at the national level; or

(iii) On the basis of the individual cumulative performance at the first, second and their MBBS examination, if such examination have been passed from the same university; or

(iv) Combination of (i) and (iii):

Provided that wherever entrance test for Postgraduate admission is held by the State Government or a university or any other authorized examining body, the minimum percentage of marks for eligibility for admission to postgraduate medical courses shall be fifty per cent for general category candidates and 40 per cent for the candidate belonging to Scheduled Castes, Scheduled Tribes and Other Backward classes.

Provided further that in non-Governmental institutions fifty percent of the total seats shall be filled by the competent authority and the remaining fifty per cent by the management of the institution on the basis of merit.

10. Period of Training

The period of training for the award of various postgraduate degrees or diplomas shall be as follows:

(1) Doctor of Medicine (M.D.) / Master of Surgery (M.S.)

The period of training for obtaining these degrees shall be three completed years including the period of examination.

Provided that in the case of students having a recognised two year postgraduate diploma course in the same subject, the period of training, including the period of examination, shall be two year.

(2) Doctor of Medicine (D.M.) / Master Chirurgiae (M.Ch.)

The period of training for obtaining these degrees shall be three completed year (including the examination period) after obtaining M.D./M.S. degrees, or equivalent recognised qualification in the required subject;

Provided that where an institution on the date of commencement for these Regulation, is imparting five year training in Neurology and Neuro-Surgery, such institution shall continue to have five year training course.

(3) Diplomas

The period of training for obtaining a postgraduate Diploma shall be two completed years including the examination period.

Migration/transfer of postgraduate student from one medical college or institution to another.

Migration/transfer of students undergoing any postgraduate course – degree /diploma shall not be permitted by any university or any authority.

Examinations

The examinations shall be organised on the basis of grading or marking system to evaluate and certify candidate's level of knowledge, skill and competence at the end of the training and obtaining a minimum of 50% marks in theory as well as practical separately shall be mandatory for passing the whole examination. The examination for M.S., M.D., D.M., M.Ch., shall be held at the end of 3 academic years (six academic terms) and for diploma at the end of 2 academic years (four academic terms). The academic terms shall mean six months training period. For other details please refer to Regulations.

Examinations

The examinations shall be organised on the basis of grading or marking system to evaluate and certify candidate's level of knowledge, skill and competence at the end of the training and obtaining a minimum of 50% marks in theory as well as practical separately shall be mandatory for passing the whole examination. The examination for M.S., M.D., D.M., M.Ch., shall be held at the end of 3 academic years (six academic terms) and for diploma at the end of 2 academic years (four academic terms). The academic terms shall mean six months training period.

For other details please refer to Regulations.

SCHEDULE

Specialities / Subjects in which Postgraduate Degree and Diploma can be awarded by the Indian Universities and the eligibility requirements of candidates for registration for the same.

A. M.D. (DOCTOR OF MEDICINE) for which candidates must possess recognised degree of MBBS (or its equivalent recognised degree)

1. Anesthesiology
2. Aviation Medicine
3. Anatomy
4. Biochemistry
5. Biophysics
6. Community Medicine
7. Dermatology, Venerology and Leprosy
8. Family Medicine
9. Forensic Medicine
10. General Medicine
11. Geriatrics
12. Health Administration
13. Hospital Administration
14. Immuno Haematology and Blood Transfusion
15. Medical Genetics
16. Microbiology
17. Nuclear Medicine
18. Pathology
19. Paediatrics
20. Pharmacology

21. Physical Medicine Rehabilitation
22. Physiology
23. Psychiatry
24. Radio-diagnosis
25. Radio-therapy
26. Rheumatology
27. Sports Medicine
28. Tropical Medicine
29. Tuberculosis & Respiratory Medicine or Pulmonary Medicine.

B. M.S. (MASTER OF SURGERY) for which candidates must possess recognised degree of MBBS (or its equivalent recognised degree).

1. Otorhinolaryngology
2. General Surgery
3. Ophthalmology
4. Orthopedics
5. Obstetrics & Gynecology

C. D.M. (DOCTOR OF MEDICINE) for which candidates must possess recognised degree of M.D. (or its equivalent recognised degree) in the subject shown against them.

D. M.Ch. (MASTER OF CHIRURGIE) for which candidates must possess recognised degree of M.S. (or its equivalent recognised degree) in the subjects shown against them.

E. Ph.D. (DOCTOR OF PHILOSOPHY)

Ph.D. Degree may be instituted in all subjects wherever recognised postgraduate qualification in medical subjects are awarded by the concerned Universities subject to fulfillment of the following guidelines :

1. Ph.D. shall be awarded only upon completion of M.D. or M.S. or P.G. Diploma or M.Sc. in medical subjects.
2. The period of training for Ph.D. shall be two years for candidates who possess M.D./M.S/P.G./ diploma in three years for candidates with M.Sc. (medical subjects).
3. For starting Ph.D. course, the institution concerned shall have the following facilities namely :-
   (i) Adequate facilities for experimental medicine and experimental surgery ;
   (ii) Ancillary Departments, adequately equipped and well staffed as prescribed for Postgraduate departments;
   (iii) Adequate facilities for advanced research work and laboratory investigations in the departments of Biochemistry, Physiology, Microbiology, Histopathology, Radio-diagnosis etc.
4. A guide for the Ph.D. degree shall have not less than fifteen year's teaching and research experience after obtaining his postgraduate qualification and shall also have not less than ten years postgraduate teaching experience as an faculty member

F. DIPLOMAS for which candidates must possess recognised degree of MBBS (or its equivalent recognised degree).

1. Anesthesiology (D.A.)
2. Clinical Pathology (D.C.P.)

3. Community Medicine (D.C.M.)
4. Dermatology, Venerology and Leprosy (DDVL)
5. Forensic Medicine (D.F.M.)
6. Health Education (D.H.E.)
7. Health Administration (D.H.A.)
8. Immuno-Haematology & Blood Transfusion (D.I.H.B.T.)
9. Marine Medicine (Dip. M.M.)
10. Microbiology (D.Micro)
11. Nutrition (D.N.)
12. Obstetrics & Gynecology (D.G.O.)
13. Occupational Health (D.O.H.)
14. Ophthalmology (D.O.)
15. Orthopedics (D.Ortho.)
16. Oto-Rhino0Laryngology(D.L.O.)
17. Paediatrics(D.C.H.)
18. Physical Medicine & Rehabilitation (D.Phy. Med. & R.)
19. Psychiatry (D.P.M.)
20. Public Health (D.P.H.)
21. Radio-diagnosis (D.M.R.D.)
22. Radio-therapy (D.M.R.T.)
23. Radiological Physics (D.R.P.)
24. Sport Medicine (D.S.M.)
25. Tropical Medicine & Health (D.T.M. & H.)
26. Tuberculosis & Chest Diseases (D.T.C.D.)
27. Virology (D.Vir.)
28. Radiation Medicine (D.R.M.)

G. DIPLOMAS for which candidates must possess recognised postgraduate degree (or its equivalent recognised degree).

1. Neuro-pathology (DNP) (with the prior requirement of M.D. (Pathology)

Code of Ethics Regulations, 2002(Published in Part III, Section 4 of the Gazette of India, dated 6th April,2002)

MEDICAL COUNCIL OF INDIA

NOTIFICATION

New Delhi, dated 11th March, 2002

No. MCI-211(2)/2001/Registration. In exercise of the powers conferred under section 20A read with section 33(m) of the Indian Medical Council Act, 1956 (102 of 1956), the Medical Council of India, with the previous approval of the Central Government, hereby makes the following regulations relating to the Professional Conduct, Etiquette and Ethics for registered medical practitioners, namely:-

Short Title and Commencement

1. These Regulations may be called the Indian Medical Council (Professional conduct, Etiquette and Ethics) Regulations, 2002.
2. They shall come into force on the date of their publication in the Official Gazette.

I. CODE OF MEDICAL ETHICS

A. Declaration

Each applicant, at the time of making an application for registration under the provisions of the Act, shall be provided a copy of the declaration and shall submit a duly signed Declaration as provided in Appendix 1. The applicant shall also certify that he/she had read and agreed to abide by the same.

B. Duties and Responsibilities of the Physician in General

1. Character of Physician

Doctors with qualification of MBBS or MBBS with post graduate degree/ diploma or with equivalent qualification in any medical discipline:

A physician shall uphold the dignity and honour of his profession.

The prime object of the medical profession is to render service to humanity; reward or financial gain is a subordinate consideration. Who- so-ever chooses his profession, assumes the obligation to conduct himself in accordance with its ideals. A physician should be an upright man, instructed in the art of healings. He shall keep himself pure in character and be diligent in caring for the sick; he should be modest, sober, patient, prompt in discharging his duty without anxiety; conducting himself with propriety in his profession and in all the actions of his life.

No person other than a doctor having qualification recognised by Medical Council of India and registered with Medical Council of India/State Medical Council (s) is allowed to practice Modern system of Medicine or Surgery. A person obtaining qualification in any other system of Medicine is not allowed to practice Modern system of Medicine in any form.

2. Maintaining Good Medical Practice

The Principal objective of the medical profession is to render service to humanity with full respect for the dignity of profession and man. Physicians should merit the confidence of patients entrusted to their care, rendering to each a full measure of service and devotion. Physicians should try continuously to improve medical knowledge and skills and should make available to their patients and colleagues the benefits of their professional attainments. The physician should practice methods of healing founded on scientific basis and should not associate professionally with anyone who violates this principle. The honoured ideals of the medical profession imply that the responsibilities of the physician extend not only to individuals but also to society.

Membership in Medical Society: For the advancement of his profession, a physician should affiliate with associations and societies of allopathic medical professions and involve actively in the functioning of such bodies.

A Physician should participate in professional meetings as part of Continuing Medical Education programmes, for at least 30 hours every five years, organized by reputed professional academic bodies or any other authorized organisaticns. The compliance of this requirement shall be informed regularly to Medical Council of India or the State Medical Councils as the case may be.

3. Maintenance of Medical Records

Every physician shall maintain the medical records pertaining to his / her indoor patients for a period of 3 years from the date of commencement of the treatment in a standard proforma laid down by the Medical Council of India and attached as Appendix 3.

If any request is made for medical records either by the patients / authorised attendant or legal authorities involved, the same may be duly acknowledged and documents shall be issued within the period of 72 hours.

A Registered medical practitioner shall maintain a Register of Medical Certificates giving full details of certificates issued. When issuing a medical certificate he /

she shall always enter the identification marks of the patient and keep a copy of the certificate. He / She shall not omit to record the signature and/or thumb mark, address and at least one identification mark of the patient on the medical certificates or report. The medical certificate shall be prepared as in Appendix 2.

Efforts shall be made to computerize medical records for quick retrieval.

4. Display of Registration Numbers

Every physician shall display the registration number accorded to him by the State Medical Council / Medical Council of India in his clinic and in all his prescriptions, certificates, money receipts given to his patients.

Physicians shall display as suffix to their names only recognized medical degrees or such certificates/diplomas and memberships/honours which confer professional knowledge or recognizes any exemplary qualification/ achievements.

5. Use of Generic Names of Drugs

Every physician should, as far as possible, prescribe drugs with generic names and he / she shall ensure that there is a rational prescription and use of drugs.

6. Highest Quality Assurance in Patient Care

Every physician should aid in safeguarding the profession against admission to it of those who are deficient in moral character or education. Physician shall not employ in connection with his professional practice any attendant who is neither registered nor enlisted under the Medical Acts in force and shall not permit such persons to attend, treat or perform operations upon patients wherever professional discretion or skill is required.

7. Exposure of Unethical Conduct

A Physician should expose, without fear or favour, incompetent or corrupt, dishonest or unethical conduct on the part of members of the profession.

8. Payment of Professional Services

The physician, engaged in the practice of medicine shall give priority to the interests of patients. The personal financial interests of a physician should not conflict with the medical interests of patients. A physician should announce his fees before rendering service and not after the operation or treatment is under way. Remuneration received for such services should be in the form and amount specifically announced to the patient at the time the service is rendered. It is unethical to enter into a contract of "no cure no payment". Physician rendering service on behalf of the state shall refrain from anticipating or accepting any consideration.

9. Evasion of Legal Restrictions

The physician shall observe the laws of the country in regulating the practice of medicine and shall also not assist others to evade such laws. He should be cooperative in observance and enforcement of sanitary laws and regulations in the interest of public health. A physician should observe the provisions of the State Acts like Drugs and Cosmetics Act, 1940; Pharmacy Act, 1948; Narcotic Drugs and Psychotropic substances Act, 1985; Medical Termination of Pregnancy Act, 1971; Transplantation of Human Organ Act, 1994; Mental Health Act, 1987; Environmental Protection Act, 1986; Pre–natal Sex Determination Test Act, 1994; Drugs and Magic Remedies (Objectionable Advertisement) Act, 1954; Persons with Disabilities (Equal Opportunities and Full Participation) Act, 1995 and Bio-Medical Waste (Management and Handling) Rules, 1998 and such other Acts, Rules, Regulations made by the Central/State

Governments or local Administrative Bodies or any other relevant Act relating to the protection and promotion of public health.

II. DUTIES OF PHYSICIANS TO THEIR PATIENTS

1. Obligations to the Sick

Though a physician is not bound to treat each and every person asking his services, he should not only be ever ready to respond to the calls of the sick and the injured, but should be mindful of the high character of his mission and the responsibility he discharges in the course of his professional duties. In his treatment, he should never forget that the health and the lives of those entrusted to his care depend on his skill and attention. A physician should endeavour to add to the comfort of the sick by making his visits at the hour indicated to the patients. A physician advising a patient to seek service of another physician is acceptable, however, in case of emergency a physician must treat the patient. No physician shall arbitrarily refuse treatment to a patient. However for good reason, when a patient is suffering from an ailment which is not within the range of experience of the treating physician, the physician may refuse treatment and refer the patient to another physician.

Medical practitioner having any incapacity detrimental to the patient or which can affect his performance vis-à-vis the patient is not permitted to practice his profession

2. Patience, Delicacy and Secrecy

Patience and delicacy should characterize the physician. Confidences concerning individual or domestic life entrusted by patients to a physician and defects in the disposition or character of patients observed during medical attendance should never be revealed unless their revelation is required by the laws of the State. Sometimes, however, a physician must determine whether his duty to society requires him to employ knowledge, obtained through confidence as a physician, to protect a healthy person against a communicable disease to which he is about to be exposed. In such instance, the physician should act as he would wish another to act toward one of his own family in like circumstances.

3. Prognosis

The physician should neither exaggerate nor minimize the gravity of a patient's condition. He should ensure himself that the patient, his relatives or his responsible friends have such knowledge of the patient's condition as will serve the best interests of the patient and the family.

4. The Patient Must Not be Neglected

A physician is free to choose whom he will serve. He should, however, respond to any request for his assistance in an emergency. Once having undertaken a case, the physician should not neglect the patient, nor should he withdraw from the case without giving adequate notice to the patient and his family. Provisionally or fully registered medical practitioner shall not willfully commit an act of negligence that may deprive his patient or patients from necessary medical care.

5. Engagement for an Obstetric Case

When a physician who has been engaged to attend an obstetric case is absent and another is sent for and delivery accomplished, the acting physician is entitled to his professional fees, but should secure the patient's consent to resign on the arrival of the physician engaged.

III. DUTIES OF PHYSICIAN IN CONSULTATION

1. Unnecessary Consultations Should be Avoided

However in case of serious illness and in doubtful or difficult conditions, the physician should request consultation, but under any circumstances such consultation should be justifiable and in the interest of the patient only and not for any other consideration.

Consulting pathologists /radiologists or asking for any other diagnostic Lab investigation should be done judiciously and not in a routine manner.

2. Consultation for Patient's Benefit

In every consultation, the benefit to the patient is of foremost importance. All physicians engaged in the case should be frank with the patient and his attendants.

3. Punctuality in Consultation

Utmost punctuality should be observed by a physician in making themselves available for consultations.

4. Statement to Patient after Consultation

All statements to the patient or his representatives should take place in the presence of the consulting physicians, except as otherwise agreed. The disclosure of the opinion to the patient or his relatives or friends shall rest with the medical attendant.

Differences of opinion should not be divulged unnecessarily but when there is irreconcilable difference of opinion the circumstances should be frankly and impartially explained to the patient or his relatives or friends. It would be opened to them to seek further advice as they so desire.

5. Treatment after Consultation

No decision should restrain the attending physician

from making such subsequent variations in the treatment if any unexpected change occurs, but at the next consultation, reasons for the variations should be discussed/explained. The same privilege, with its obligations, belongs to the consultant when sent for in an emergency during the absence of attending physician. The attending physician may prescribe medicine at any time for the patient, whereas the consultant may prescribe only in case of emergency or as an expert when called for.

6. Patients Referred to Specialists

When a patient is referred to a specialist by the attending physician, a case summary of the patient should be given to the specialist, who should communicate his opinion in writing to the attending physician.

7. Fees and Other Charges

A physician shall clearly display his fees and other charges on the board of his chamber and/or the hospitals he is visiting. Prescription should also make clear if the Physician himself dispensed any medicine.

A physician shall write his name and designation in full along with registration particulars in his prescription letter head.

Note: In Government hospital where the patient–load is heavy, the name of the prescribing doctor must be written below his/her signature.

IV. RESPONSIBILITIES OF PHYSICIANS TO EACH OTHER

A physician should consider it as a pleasure and privilege to render gratuitous service to all physicians and their immediate family dependants.

Conduct in Consultation

In consultations, no insincerity, rivalry or envy should be indulged in. All due respect should be observed towards the physician in-charge of the case and no statement or remark be made, which would impair the confidence reposed in him. For this purpose no discussion should be carried on in the presence of the patient or his representatives.

Consultant Not to Take Charge of the Case

When a physician has been called for consultation, the Consultant should normally not take charge of the case, especially on the solicitation of the patient or friends. The Consultant shall not criticize the referring physician. He / she shall discuss the diagnosis treatment plan with the referring physician.

Appointment of Substitute

Whenever a physician requests another physician to attend his patients during his temporary absence from his practice, professional courtesy requires the acceptance of such appointment only when he has the capacity to discharge the additional responsibility along with his / her other duties. The physician acting under such an appointment should give the utmost consideration to the interests and reputation of the absent physician and all such patients should be restored to the care of the latter upon his/her return.

Visiting Another Physician's Case

When it becomes the duty of a physician occupying an official position to see and report upon an illness or injury, he should communicate to the physician in attendance so as to give him an option of being present. The medical officer / physician occupying an official position should avoid remarks upon the diagnosis or the treatment that has been adopted.

V. DUTIES OF PHYSICIAN TO THE PUBLIC AND TO THE PARAMEDICAL PROFESSION

1. Physicians as Citizens

Physicians, as good citizens, possessed of special training should disseminate advice on public health issues. They should play their part in enforcing the laws of the community and in sustaining the institutions that advance the interests of humanity. They should particularly co-operate with the authorities in the administration of sanitary/public health laws and regulations.

2. Public and Community Health

Physicians, especially those engaged in public health work, should enlighten the public concerning quarantine regulations and measures for the prevention of epidemic and communicable diseases. At all times the physician should notify the constituted public health authorities of every case of communicable disease under his care, in accordance with the laws, rules and regulations of the health authorities. When an epidemic occurs a physician should not abandon his duty for fear of contracting the disease himself.

3. Pharmacists / Nurses

Physicians should recognize and promote the practice of different paramedical services such as, pharmacy and nursing as professions and should seek their cooperation wherever required.

VI. UNETHICAL ACTS

A physician shall not aid or abet or commit any of the following acts which shall be construed as unethical -

1. Advertising

Soliciting of patients directly or indirectly, by a physician, by a group of physicians or by institutions or organisations is unethical. A physician shall not make use of him / her (or his / her name) as subject of any form or manner of advertising or publicity through any mode either alone or in conjunction with others which is of such a character as to invite attention to him or to his professional position, skill, qualification, achievements, attainments, specialities, appointments, associations, affiliations or honours and/or of such character as would ordinarily result in his self aggrandizement. A physician shall not give to any person, whether for compensation or otherwise, any approval, recommendation, endorsement, certificate, report or statement with respect of any drug, medicine, nostrum remedy, surgical, or therapeutic article, apparatus or appliance or any commercial product or article with respect of any property, quality or use thereof or any test, demonstration or trial thereof, for use in connection with his name, signature, or photograph in any form or manner of advertising through any mode nor shall he boast of cases, operations, cures or remedies or permit the publication of report thereof through any mode. A medical practitioner is however permitted to make a formal announcement in press regarding the following:

1. On starting practice.
2. On change of type of practice.
3. On changing address.
4. On temporary absence from duty.
5. On resumption of another practice.
6. On succeeding to another practice.
7. Public declaration of charges.

Printing of self photograph, or any such material of publicity in the letter head or on sign board of the consulting room or any such clinical establishment shall be regarded as acts of self advertisement and unethical conduct on the part of the physician. However, printing of sketches, diagrams, picture of human system shall not be treated as unethical.

2. Patent and Copy rights

A physician may patent surgical instruments, appliances and medicine or Copyright applications, methods and procedures. However, it shall be unethical if the benefits of such patents or copyrights are not made available in situations where the interest of large population is involved.

3. Running an Open Shop (Dispensing of Drugs and Appliances by Physicians)

A physician should not run an open shop for sale of medicine for dispensing prescriptions prescribed by doctors other than himself or for sale of medical or surgical appliances. It is not unethical for a physician to prescribe or supply drugs, remedies or appliances as long as there is no exploitation of the patient. Drugs prescribed by a physician or brought from the market for a patient should explicitly state the proprietary formulae as well as generic name of the drug.

4. Rebates and Commission

A physician shall not give, solicit, or receive nor shall he offer to give solicit or receive, any gift, gratuity, commission or bonus in consideration of or return for the referring, recommending or procuring of any patient for medical, surgical or other treatment. A physician shall not directly or indirectly, participate in or be a party to act of division, transference, assignment, subordination, rebating, splitting or refunding of any fee for medical, surgical or other treatment.

Provisions of para 6.4.1 shall apply with equal force to the referring, recommending or procuring by a physician or any person, specimen or material for diagnostic purposes or other study / work. Nothing in this section, however, shall prohibit payment of salaries by a qualified physician to other duly qualified person rendering medical care under his supervision.

5. Secret Remedies

The prescribing or dispensing by a physician of secret remedial agents of which he does not know the composition, or the manufacture or promotion of their use is unethical and as such prohibited. All the drugs prescribed by a physician should always carry a proprietary formula and clear name.

6. Human Rights

The physician shall not aid or abet torture nor shall he be a party to either infliction of mental or physical trauma or concealment of torture inflicted by some other person or agency in clear violation of human rights.

7. Euthanasia

Practicing euthanasia shall constitute unethical conduct. However on specific occasion, the question of withdrawing supporting devices to sustain cardio-pulmonary function even after brain death, shall be decided only by a team of doctors and not merely by the treating physician alone. A team of doctors shall declare withdrawal of support system. Such team shall consist of the doctor in charge of the patient, Chief Medical Officer / Medical Officer in charge of the hospital and a doctor nominated by the in-charge of the hospital from the hospital staff or in accordance with the provisions of the Transplantation of Human Organ Act, 1994.

VII. MISCONDUCT

The following acts of commission or omission on the part of

a physician shall constitute professional misconduct rendering him/her liable for disciplinary action:

1. Violation of the Regulations: If he/she commits any violation of these Regulations.
2. If he/she does not maintain the medical records of his/her indoor patients for a period of three years as per regulation 1.3 and refuses to provide the same within 72 hours when the patient or his/her authorised representative makes a request for it as per the regulation 1.3.2.
3. If he/she does not display the registration number accorded to him/her by the State Medical Council or the Medical Council of India in his clinic, prescriptions and certificates etc. issued by him or violates the provisions of regulation 1.4.2.
4. Adultery or Improper Conduct: Abuse of professional position by committing adultery or improper conduct with a patient or by maintaining an improper association with a patient will render a Physician liable for disciplinary action as provided under the Indian Medical Council Act, 1956 or the concerned State Medical Council Act.
5. Conviction by Court of Law: Conviction by a Court of Law for offences involving moral turpitude / Criminal acts.
6. Sex Determination Tests: On no account sex determination test shall be undertaken with the intent to terminate the life of a female foetus developing in her mother's womb, unless there are other absolute indications for termination of pregnancy as specified in the Medical Termination of Pregnancy Act, 1971. Any act of termination of pregnancy of normal female foetus amounting to

female foeticide shall be regarded as professional misconduct on the part of the physician leading to penal erasure besides rendering him liable to criminal proceedings as per the provisions of this Act.

7. Signing Professional Certificates, Reports and other Documents: Registered medical practitioners are in certain cases bound by law to give, or may from time to time be called upon or requested to give certificates, notification, reports and other documents of similar character signed by them in their professional capacity for subsequent use in the courts or for administrative purposes etc. Such documents, among others, include the ones given at Appendix – 4. Any registered practitioner who is shown to have signed or given under his name and authority any such certificate, notification, report or document of a similar character which is untrue, misleading or improper, is liable to have his name deleted from the Register.

8. A registered medical practitioner shall not contravene the provisions of the Drugs and Cosmetics Act and regulations made there under. Accordingly,

   (a) Prescribing steroids/ psychotropic drugs when there is no absolute medical indication;

   (b) selling Schedule 'H' & 'L' drugs and poisons to the public except to his patient;

   in contravention of the above provisions shall constitute gross professional misconduct on the part of the physician.

9. Performing or enabling unqualified person to perform an abortion or any illegal operation for which there is no medical, surgical or psychological indication.

10. A registered medical practitioner shall not issue

certificates of efficiency in modern medicine to unqualified or non-medical person.

Note: The foregoing does not restrict the proper training and instruction of bonafide students, midwives, dispensers, surgical attendants, or skilled mechanical and technical assistants and therapy assistants under the personal supervision of physicians.

11. A physician should not contribute to the lay press articles and give interviews regarding diseases and treatments which may have the effect of advertising himself or soliciting practices; but is open to write to the lay press under his own name on matters of public health, hygienic living or to deliver public lectures, give talks on the radio/TV/internet chat for the same purpose and send announcement of the same to lay press.

12. An institution run by a physician for a particular purpose such as a maternity home, nursing home, private hospital, rehabilitation centre or any type of training institution etc. may be advertised in the lay press, but such advertisements should not contain anything more than the name of the institution, type of patients admitted, type of training and other facilities offered and the fees.

13. It is improper for a physician to use an unusually large sign board and write on it anything other than his name, qualifications obtained from a University or a statutory body, titles and name of his speciality, registration number including the name of the State Medical Council under which registered. The same should be the contents of his prescription papers. It is improper to affix a sign-board on a chemist's shop or in places where he does not reside or work.

14. The registered medical practitioner shall not disclose the secrets of a patient that have been learnt in the exercise of his / her profession except –
    (i) in a court of law under orders of the Presiding Judge;
    (ii) in circumstances where there is a serious and identified risk to a specific person and / or community; and
    (iii) notifiable diseases.

    In case of communicable / notifiable diseases, concerned public health authorities should be informed immediately.
15. The registered medical practitioner shall not refuse on religious grounds alone to give assistance in or conduct of sterility, birth control, circumcision and medical termination of Pregnancy when there is medical indication, unless the medical practitioner feels himself/herself incompetent to do so.
16. Before performing an operation the physician should obtain in writing the consent from the husband or wife, parent or guardian in the case of minor, or the patient himself as the case may be. In an operation which may result in sterility the consent of both husband and wife is needed.
17. A registered medical practitioner shall not publish photographs or case reports of his / her patients without their permission, in any medical or other journal in a manner by which their identity could be made out. If the identity is not to be disclosed, the consent is not needed.
18. In the case of running of a nursing home by a physician and employing assistants to help him / her, the ultimate responsibility rests on the physician.

19. A Physician shall not use touts or agents for procuring patients.
20. A Physician shall not claim to be specialist unless he has a special qualification in that branch.
21. No act of invitro fertilization or artificial insemination shall be undertaken without the informed consent of the female patient and her spouse as well as the donor. Such consent shall be obtained in writing only after the patient is provided, at her own level of comprehension, with sufficient information about the purpose, methods, risks, inconveniences, disappointments of the procedure and possible risks and hazards.
22. Research: Clinical drug trials or other research involving patients or volunteers as per the guidelines of ICMR can be undertaken, provided ethical considerations are borne in mind. Violation of existing ICMR guidelines in this regard shall constitute misconduct. Consent taken from the patient for trial of drug or therapy which is not as per the guidelines shall also be construed as misconduct.
23. If a physician posted in rural area is found absent on more than two occasions during inspection by the Head of the District Health Authority or the Chairman, Zila Parishad, the same shall be construed as a misconduct if it is recommended to the Medical Council of India/State Medical Council by the State Government for action under these Regulations.
24. If a physician posted in a medical college/institution both as teaching faculty or otherwise shall remain in hospital/college during the assigned duty hours. If they are found absent on more than two occasions during this period, the same shall be construed as a

misconduct if it is certified by the Principal/Medical Superintendent and forwarded through the State Government to Medical Council of India/State Medical Council for action under these Regulations.

VIII. PUNISHMENT AND DISCIPLINARY ACTION

8.1 It must be clearly understood that the instances of offences and of Professional misconduct which are given above do not constitute and are not intended to constitute a complete list of the infamous acts which calls for disciplinary action, and that by issuing this notice the Medical Council of India and or State Medical Councils are in no way precluded from considering and dealing with any other form of professional misconduct on the part of a registered practitioner. Circumstances may and do arise from time to time in relation to which there may occur questions of professional misconduct which do not come within any of these categories. Every care should be taken that the code is not violated in letter or spirit. In such instances as in all others, the Medical Council of India and/or State Medical Councils have to consider and decide upon the facts brought before the Medical Council of India and/or State Medical Councils.

8.2 It is made clear that any complaint with regard to professional misconduct can be brought before the appropriate Medical Council for Disciplinary action. Upon receipt of any complaint of professional misconduct, the appropriate Medical Council would hold an enquiry and give opportunity to the registered medical practitioner to be heard in person or by pleader. If the medical practitioner is found to be guilty of committing professional misconduct, the appropriate Medical Council may award such punishment as deemed necessary or may direct the removal altogether or for a specified period, from the register of the name of the delinquent registered practitioner. Deletion from the Register shall be widely publicized in local press as well as in the publications of different Medical Associations/ Societies/ Bodies.

8.3 In case the punishment of removal from the register is for a limited period, the appropriate Council may also direct that the name so removed shall be restored in the register after the expiry of the period for which the name was ordered to be removed.

8.4 Decision on complaint against delinquent physician shall be taken within a time limit of 6 months.

8.5 During the pendency of the complaint the appropriate Council may restrain the physician from performing the procedure or practice which is under scrutiny.

8.6 Professional incompetence shall be judged by peer group as per guidelines prescribed by Medical Council of India.

APPENDIX – 1

DECLARATION

At the time of registration, each applicant shall be given a copy of the following declaration by the Registrar concerned and the applicant shall read and agree to abide by the same:

1. I solemnly pledge myself to consecrate my life to service of humanity.
2. Even under threat, I will not use my medical knowledge contrary to the laws of Humanity.
3. I will maintain the utmost respect for human life from the time of conception.
4. I will not permit considerations of religion, nationality, race, party politics or social standing

to intervene between my duty and my patient.

5. I will practice my profession with conscience and dignity.
6. The health of my patient will be my first consideration.
7. I will respect the secrets which are confined in me.
8. I will give to my teachers the respect and gratitude which is their due.
9. I will maintain by all means in my power, the honour and noble traditions of medical profession.
10. I will treat my colleagues with all respect and dignity.
11. I shall abide by the code of medical ethics as enunciated in the Indian Medical Council (Professional Conduct, Etiquette and Ethics) Regulations 2002.

I make these promises solemnly, freely and upon my honour.

Signature ....

Name ....

Place ....

Address

....

....

....

Date ....

APPENDIX – 2

FORM OF CERTIFICATE RECOMMENDED FOR LEAVE OR EXTENSION OR COMMUNICATION OF LEAVE AND FOR FITNESS

Signature of patient or thumb impression ....
To be filled in by the applicant in the presence of the Government Medical Attendant, or Medical Practitioner.

Identification marks:-

1. ....

2. ....

I, Dr. ____________________________ after careful examination of the case certify hereby that ________________ whose signature is given above is suffering from ____________________ and I consider that a period of absence from duty of ______________ with effect from ______________ is absolutely necessary for the restoration of his health.

I, Dr. ________________________ after careful examination of the case certify hereby that ____________________ on restoration of health is now fit to join service.

Place ______________________ Signature of Medical attendant.

Date ________________________ Registration No. ____________

(Medical Council of India / State Medical Council of .... State)

Note: The nature and probable duration of the illness should also be specified. This certificate must be accompanied by a brief resume of the case giving the nature of the illness, its symptoms, causes and duration.

APPENDIX – 3

FORMAT FOR MEDICAL RECORD

(See Regulation 3.1)

Name of the patient: ______________________

Age : ______________________

Sex : ______________________

Address : ______________________

Occupation : ______________________

Date of 1st visit : ______________________

Clinical note (summary) of the case: ______________________

Prov. : Diagnosis : ______________________

Investigations advised with reports:

Diagnosis after investigation: ______________________

Advice : ______________________

Follow up Date: ______________________

Observations: ______________________

Signature in full ______________________

Name of Treating Physician

____

____

APPENDIX – 4

LIST OF CERTIFICATES, REPORTS, NOTIFICATIONS ETC. ISSUED BY DOCTORS FOR THE PURPOSES OF VARIOUS ACTS / ADMINISTRATIVE REQUIREMENTS

(a) Under the acts relating to birth, death or disposal of the dead.

(b) Under the Acts relating to Lunacy and Mental Deficiency and under the Mental illness Act and the rules made thereunder.

(c) Under the Vaccination Acts and the regulations made thereunder.

(d) Under the Factory Acts and the regulations made thereunder.

(e) Under the Education Acts.

(f) Under the Public Health Acts and the orders made thereunder.

(g) Under the Workmen's Compensation Act and Persons with Disability Act.

(h) Under the Acts and orders relating to the notification of infectious diseases.

(i) Under the Employee's State Insurance Act.

(j) In connection with sick benefit insurance and friendly societies.

(k) Under the Merchant Shipping Act.

(l) For procuring / issuing of passports.

(m) For excusing attendance in courts of Justice, in public services, in public offices or in ordinary employment.

(n) In connection with Civil and Military matters.

(o) In connection with matters under the control of Department of Pensions.

(p) In connection with quarantine rules.

(q) For procuring driving licence.

(DR. M. SACHDEVA)
SECRETARY
MEDICAL COUNCIL OF INDIA

2

Rules for Hospital and Health Services

The Acts of 2000

AN ACT RELATIVE TO HALE HOSPITAL IN THE CITY OF HAVERHILL

Be it enacted by the Senate and House of Representatives in General Court assembled, and by the authority of the same, as follows:

Section 1

Chapter 569 of the acts of 1985 is hereby amended by striking out section 1 and inserting in place thereof the following three sections:-

Section 1. For the purposes of this act the following words shall have the following meanings:-

"Board", the board of trustees of the Hale hospital.

"City", the city of Haverhill.

"City council", the city council of the city of Haverhill.

"Health care purchaser", an entity licensed or authorized to do business in the commonwealth under chapter 175 of the General Laws, organised under chapter 176A, 176B or 176G of the General Laws; approved under chapter 176I of the General Laws, a health plan purchasing cooperative, or any other entity that enters into arrangements with health care providers to provide services on behalf of a defined population.

"Hospital", the Hale hospital.

"Mayor", the mayor of the city of Haverhill.

"Medical practice", an individual, professional corporation, limited liability company, medical group practice or similar entity that engages in providing professional medical services.

"Service area", the geographic area defined from time to time by the board as the area within which the hospital provides services. The service area may include portions of New Hampshire.

Section 1A. (a) The hospital established and maintained by the city shall be designated and known as the Hale hospital. All provisions in any special law that refers to the Hale municipal hospital, the Haverhill Hale municipal hospital, the Haverhill municipal (Hale) hospital, or similar designation shall be deemed to mean the Hale hospital. All presently existing legal rights and obligations created by statute, contract or otherwise pertaining to the hospital shall be deemed to be rights and obligations of the Hale hospital.

(b) The person who functions as chief executive officer of the Hale hospital shall be referred to as the chief executive officer. All provisions in any special law that refers to the administrator or director of Hale hospital shall be deemed to mean the chief executive officer of the Hale hospital.

Section 1B. The city of Haverhill may issue refunding bonds for the purpose of paying or refunding all or any designated part of its bond then outstanding issued under chapter 451 of the acts of 1978. Except as provided in this act the issuance of refunding bonds, the maturities and other details thereof, the security therefor, and the rights, duties and obligations of the city in respect to the same shall be governed by the applicable provisions of said chapter 451 relating to the issuance of bonds other than refunding bonds, including the provisions of section 1A of said chapter 451 relating to establishment of a hospital debt service fund. The refunding bonds may be issued in amounts sufficient to pay or provide for the payment of the principal of the bonds being refunded, together with any redemption premium thereon, any interest accrued or to accrue to the date of payment of such bonds, the cxpenses of issue of the refunding bonds and the expense of redeeming the bonds being refunded. Such refunding bonds may be issued at one time or from time to time and may be refunded by the issuance of additional refunding bonds under the act; provided, however, that no refunding bonds shall be payable over a period longer than 30 years from the date of the original bonds issued under said chapter 451. For each issue the amounts of principal and interest payable in each year shall be determined in accordance with said chapter 451 beginning with the earliest stated principal maturity date for any of the bonds being refunded. If such refunding bonds are issued prior to the maturity or redemption date of the bonds, the proceeds thereof together with other moneys then available or to become available to the city, which moneys may include income to be derived from the investment of such proceeds, sufficient to pay or provide for the payment of the principal, redemption premium, if any, and interest on the bonds so refunded to the date fixed for their payment or redemption shall be held in a separate fund and in trust solely for the payment of such principal, redemption premium and interest. The funds so held may be invested pursuant to section 55 of chapter 44 of the General Laws and the income derived from such investment may be expended to pay the principal, redemption premium, if any, and interest on the bonds being refunded until they are paid or redeemed; provided that notwithstanding any limitation on the maturity of investments under said section 55, any such investment may have a maturity not later than the date fixed for the payment or redemption of the bonds being refunded. Upon payment of the refunded bonds or establishment of a refunding trust in accordance with this section, any hospital debt service fund established under section 1A of said chapter 451 for the bonds being refunded and any trust agreement or credit agreement executed in connection with the issuance of the bonds being refunded may be terminated or modified so as to apply to and provide security for the refunding bonds; provided, however, that any moneys in such a hospital debt service fund on the date of issuance of the refunding bonds that the city treasurer determines to be unnecessary to pay debt service on the refunded bonds shall be credited to the city's unreserved general fund balance.

Section 2

Section 3 of said chapter 569 is hereby amended by striking out, in line 4, the word "one" and inserting in place thereof the following word:- 1B.

Section 3

The first paragraph of section 4 of said chapter 569 is hereby amended by striking out the fourth and fifth sentences and inserting in place thereof the following four sentences:- Except as otherwise specifically provided by this act, expenditure from the account authorized by this section shall be made by the chief executive officer of the Hale hospital, subject to appropriation in accordance with chapter 44 of the General Laws, and shall be used for the operation, maintenance, service development, capital equipment and plant for said hospital and for such other purposes as are consistent with the provisions of this act. Said account authorized by this section shall be deemed to be a trust fund. It shall be maintained and invested on behalf of said hospital by the treasurer of the city of Haverhill, and any income accruing thereon shall inure to the benefit of the hospital; provided, however, that such funds shall be invested in any investment as may be lawful for fiduciaries in the commonwealth. Notwithstanding any general or special laws to the contrary and notwithstanding the fact that expenditures from said account are subject to appropriation in accordance with this section, the chief executive officer, with the approval of the board, may transfer funds among the hospital's items of appropriation without the specific approval of the city council and may create job classifications for the hospital's personnel and establish pay scales for the positions so created; if in the aggregate, the hospital does not expend in any fiscal year an amount in excess of the amount total appropriated from the enterprise account for that year, except as may be otherwise provided by this act.

Section 4

Section 4B of said chapter 569, inserted by section 1A of chapter 58 of the acts of 1990, is hereby amended by striking out the sixth paragraph.

Section 5

Said chapter 569 is hereby further amended by inserting after section 6 the following eight sections:-

Section 6A. Subject to appropriation as required by section 4, the chief executive officer, with the approval of the board, may enter into agreements on behalf of the city and of the hospital with any medical practice to provide professional services in the hospital's service area; to facilitate the development of the hospital's medical staff; to provide management services, by itself or in conjunction with a joint venturer in accordance with the provisions of section 9 to a medical practice; to pay expenses associated with physicians relocating to the hospital's service area; to make loans, as permitted by law, to support minimum salary or the purchase of equipment for physicians relocating to the hospital's service area, provided that each physician receiving such support agrees to serve on the hospital's active medical staff for the period during which any such loan has outstanding principal or interest, that a reasonable rate of interest be charged and that such loan be on such additional reasonable terms and conditions as the board determines; and to provide such additional service supports as are determined to be reasonable by the chief executive officer and the board.

Section 6B. Subject to appropriation as required by section 4, the hospital, by vote of a majority of the full membership of the board, may make investment, hold stock in or otherwise participate in the governance of a physician/hospital organisation, independent practice association, medical service corporation or joint venture with physicians and other hospitals, regardless of the form it takes, for the purpose of developing the medical staff of the hospital and for contracting with health care purchasers to provide hospital or medical services under the terms of any health insurance plan or benefit, including for purposes of entering into contracts under the terms of which the hospital will take risk for the services provided by such arrangement. By vote of a majority of the full membership of the board in each instance the hospital may delegate to any such entity the right to negotiate and execute contracts with health care purchasers on its behalf including risk contracts and to agree to be bound by the terms of any contract so negotiated and entered into on its behalf including terms relating to the allocation of risk to the hospital through the hospital's participation in risk pools or other risk arrangements. The hospital may appoint one or more members of the board or one or more hospital or city employees to serve as members of the governing body and of committees, and as officers of any such organisation, if their participation in any such capacity is approved by the board. Such board members and employees shall not by so serving violate section 17 or section 19 of chapter 268A of the General Laws, and section 20 of said chapter 268A shall not apply with respect to any interest such board member or employee may have with regard to any contract between the city and any such organisation entered into within the scope of this section where such interest arises because of an appointment made pursuant to this section.

Section 6C. The hospital is hereby authorized to enter into joint venture arrangements with any individual, private, nonprofit, for-profit or public entity or agency to provide health care services within its service area or to engage in any activity or undertaking necessary or incidental thereto. Any such arrangement must be approved by a majority of the full membership of the board, and the chief executive officer may, pursuant to any such vote, expend funds from the hospital's enterprise account, subject to appropriation as provided in section 4, for purposes of engaging in such joint venture arrangement; provided, however, that in using its funds for such purpose the hospital shall act in a manner consistent with the regulations of the Internal Revenue Service applicable to organisations that are exempt from federal income tax under section 501(c) of the Internal Revenue Code of 1986, or a successor thereto, when such organisation is engaged in a joint venture with an entity that is not so exempt. The hospital may appoint one or more members of the board or one or more hospital or city employees to serve as members of the governing body and of committees, and as officers of any such joint venture arrangement organisation, if their participation in any such capacity is approved by the board. Such board members and employees shall not by so serving violate section 17 or section 19 of chapter 268A of the General Laws, and section 20 of said chapter 268A shall not apply with respect to any interest such board member or employee may have with regard to any contract between the city and any such organisation entered into within the scope of this section where such interest arises because of an appointment made pursuant to this section.

Section 6D. Notwithstanding any general or special laws to the contrary or the provisions of any ordinance of the city, the mayor may appoint persons who are not residents of the city to the board, but at no time shall persons who are nonresidents of the city constitute more than one-third of the full membership of the board. In appointing persons to the board who are not residents of the city, the mayor shall consider the desire to have representation on the board from cities and towns within the hospital's service area, other than the city, and from any system or systems with which the hospital is affiliated, as provided in section 6F.

Section 6E. Notwithstanding any general or special law to the contrary, the hospital may develop health care services in locations anywhere within its service area, including outside of the city, and may expend funds from the hospital's enterprise account for this purpose, including, as deemed appropriate by the board and as authorized by an appropriation approved pursuant to section 4 acquiring or leasing real estate for such purposes, if the development of such services does not jeopardize the hospital's principal mission of promoting health care services for the residents of the city.

Section 6F. (a) By vote of a majority of the full membership of the board and the approval of the city council, the hospital may enter into affiliation arrangements with one or more health care systems, each of which includes one or more other hospitals that are formed for purposes that include, but are not limited to, coordinating more effective provision of health care services and undertaking more effective contracting with managed care plans. For purposes of this section, "affiliation arrangements" shall mean the creation of a relationship whereby the hospital participates as a component of the broader health care system including, subject to other provisions of this section, participation in the governance of such system, in managed care risk and other third party payor contracts negotiated on behalf of such system, and in joint strategic, business and financial planning within such system. Subject to appropriation pursuant to section 4, the hospital may expend amounts in its enterprise account in furtherance of the common purposes of a system with which it affiliates.

(b) In conjunction with any system with which the hospital enters into an affiliation arrangement in accordance with this section, by vote of a majority of the full membership of the board in each instance, the hospital may delegate to an entity within such system the right to negotiate and execute contracts with health care purchasers on its behalf, including risk contracts, and to agree to be bound by the terms of any contract so negotiated and entered into on behalf of the system, including terms relating to the allocation of risk to the hospital through the hospital's participation in risk pools or other risk arrangements.

(c) In conjunction with any system with which the

hospital enters into an affiliation arrangement in accordance with this section, the hospital may serve as a member of any nonprofit organisation that is a part of such system or as a shareholder or member of any for-profit entity or limited liability company that is part of such system. The hospital may appoint one or more members of the board or one or more hospital or city employees to serve as members of the governing body and of committees, and as officers of any constituent entity or entities included within any such system, if the participation of any such person in any such capacity is approved by the board and by the mayor. Such board members and employees shall not by so serving violate section 17 or section 19 of chapter 268A of the General Laws, and section 20 of said chapter 268A shall not apply with respect to any interest such board member or employee may have with regard to any contract between the city and any such organisation entered into within the scope of this section.where such interest arises because of an appointment made pursuant to this section.

(d)This section shall be deemed to provide a complete, additional and alternative method for the effectuation of the purposes of this section and shall be construed to be supplemental to, and not in derogation of, powers otherwise conferred by law; but insofar as this section is inconsistent with any general or special law, administrative order or regulation or any limitation imposed by the municipal charter of the city, this section shall be controlling. This section shall be interpreted liberally to effectuate its purposes.

Section 6G. (a) For purposes of this section, "authorized officers" shall mean the mayor, the city auditor and the chairman of the hospital board, acting unanimously; but each of said individuals may designate any other officer of the city, or, in the case of the chairman of the board, the chief executive officer, to act on his behalf as an authorized officer for any and all purposes under this section. For purposes of this definition, "officer of the city" shall mean a person who is in charge of a department of the city or who is a member of an administrative board of the city. The mayor, city auditor and chairman of the hospital board shall not all designate the same person to serve as an authorized officer, nor shall any two of them designate the same person so to serve.

(b) The city may provide for the issuance from time to time of debt obligations on behalf of the hospital for any of its purposes. Any borrowing by the city on behalf of the hospital under the provisions of this section shall be subject to authorisation by a two-thirds vote of the city council, with the approval of the mayor. All such debt obligations shall be negotiable for all purposes without regard to any other law subject only to the provisions of any such debt obligations for registration.

(c) Debt obligations issued under this section may be secured by a pledge, mortgage of or security interest in any and all assets of the hospital, whether real or personal, tangible or intangible, whether then existing or thereafter arising, including but not limited to revenues, receipts, cash, accounts, goods, equipment, inventory, general intangibles, securities or other assets or funds of the hospital, by mortgages or other instruments covering all or any part of the foregoing, including any additions, improvements, extensions to or enlargements of any real property thereafter made, or by any one or more of the foregoing, all as may be determined by the authorized officers. Debt obligations may be dated, may bear interest at such rate or rates, including rates variable from time to time, may be payable in any domestic or foreign currency and at any domestic or foreign location and may mature or otherwise be payable at such time or times as may be provided for by the authorized officers, and may be made redeemable or determinable prior to maturity at the option of the hospital or the holder thereof at such price or prices and under such terms and conditions as may be fixed by the authorized officers.

(d) The authorized officers shall determine the form of debt obligations and the manner of execution, denomination or denominations and place or places of payment thereof. In case any officer whose signature or a facsimile of whose signature shall appear on any debt obligations shall cease to be such officer before the delivery thereof, such signature or such facsimile shall nevertheless be valid and sufficient for all purposes as if such officer had remained in office until after such delivery. The authorized officers may provide for the authentication of debt obligations by a trustee, fiscal agent, registrar or transfer agent.

(e) In the discretion of the authorized officers, debt obligations of the city issued under this section may be issued with such terms as will cause the interest thereon to be subject to federal income taxation. The city may sell the hospital's debt obligations in such manner, either at public or private sale, for such price, at such rate or rates of interest, or at discount in lieu of interest, as the authorized officers determine will best effectuate its corporate purposes.

(f) In the discretion of the city council, any debt obligations issued hereunder may be secured by a resolution of the city council or by a trust agreement between the city, on behalf of the hospital, and the Massachusetts Health and Educational Facilities authority established by chapter 614 of the acts of 1968 and, for this purpose, the hospital shall be deemed to be a hospital within the meaning of section 3 of said chapter 614, or a corporate trustee, which corporate trustee may be any trust company or bank having the powers of a trust company within or without the commonwealth, and any such trust agreement shall be in such form and executed in such manner as may be determined by the authorized officers. Such trust agreement or resolution may pledge or assign, in whole or in part, any revenues, receipts, cash, accounts, inventory, general intangibles, or other assets and funds, held or to be received by the hospital, and its real property, including any additions, improvements, extensions to or enlargements of any real property thereafter made, and any contract or other rights to receive the same, whether then existing or thereafter coming into existence and whether then held or thereafter acquired by the hospital, and the proceeds thereof. Such trust agreement or resolution may contain such provisions for protecting and enforcing the rights, security and remedies of holders of debt obligations as may be reasonable or advisable, including, without limiting the generality of the foregoing, provisions defining defaults and providing for remedies in the event thereof, which may include the acceleration of maturities, restrictions on individual right of action by holders of debt obligations and covenants setting forth duties of and limitations on the hospital in relation to the conduct of its programs and the management of its property, the custody, safeguarding, investment and application of moneys, the issuance of additional or refunding debt obligations, the establishment of reserves and the making and amending of contracts.

(g) In addition to other security provided in this act or otherwise by law, debt obligations issued by the city under this section may be secured, in whole or in part, by financial guaranties, by insurance or by letters of credit issued to the city or the hospital, or a trustee, or any other person by any bank, trust company, insurance or surety company or other financial institution, within or without the commonwealth, and the city may pledge or assign any and all assets of the hospital, whether then existing or thereafter arising, including but not limited to revenues, receipts, cash, accounts, goods, equipment, inventory, general intangibles, securities, or other assets and funds of the hospital, including any additions, improvements, extensions to or enlargements of any real property thereafter made, as security for such guaranties or insurance or for the reimbursement by the city to the issuer of any such letter of credit of any payments made under such letter of credit.

(h) It shall be lawful for any bank or trust company to act as a depository or trustee of the proceeds of debt obligations, revenues or other moneys under any trust agreement or resolution provided for herein and to furnish such indemnification or to pledge such securities and issue such letters of credit as may be required by the city. Any such trust agreement or resolution may set forth the rights and remedies of holders of debt obligations and of the trustee and may restrict the individual right of action by holders of debt obligations. Any pledge of hospital revenues or other property made by the city under the provisions of this section, including, without limitation, any pledge by the city of its rights to receive payments of any kind from or for the account of mortgagors under mortgages, participations therein or subsidy, guaranty, insurance or other contracts relating thereto, and of its revenues and other property, and of the mortgages, notes, such participations, such subsidy, guaranty, insurance or other contracts or other collateral, and of the proceeds of any or all thereof shall be valid and binding and shall be deemed continuously perfected for the purposes of chapter 106 of the General Laws and other laws from the time when such pledge is made. The revenues, moneys, property, rights and proceeds so pledged and then held or thereafter acquired or received by the city or the hospital shall immediately be subject to the lien of such pledge without any physical delivery or segregation thereof or further act, and the lien of any such pledge shall be valid and binding against all parties having claims of any kind in tort, contract or otherwise against the city or the hospital, regardless of whether such parties have notice thereof. Neither the resolution, any trust agreement nor any other agreement by which a pledge is created need be filed or recorded except in the records of the city, and no filing need be made under said chapter 106 or any other law.

(i) Any holder of a debt obligation issued by the city under the provisions of this section and any trustee under a trust agreement or resolution securing the same, except to the extent the rights herein given may be restricted by such trust agreement or resolution, may bring suit upon the debt obligations and may, either at law or in equity, by suit, action, mandamus or other proceeding for legal or equitable relief, including proceedings for the appointment of a receiver to take possession and control of the business and properties of the hospital, to operate and maintain the same, to make any necessary repair, renewals and replacements in respect thereof and to fix, revise and collect fees and charges, protect and enforce any and all rights under the laws of the commonwealth or granted hereunder or under such trust agreement, resolution or other agreement and may enforce and compel the performance of all duties required by this section or by such trust agreement or resolution to be performed by the city, the hospital or by any officer thereof.

(j) Debt obligations issued by the city under this section are hereby made securities in which all public officers and public bodies of the commonwealth and its political subdivisions, all insurance companies, trust companies in their commercial departments, savings banks, cooperative banks, banking associations, investment companies, executors, administrators, trustees and other fiduciaries may properly and legally invest funds, including capital in their control or belonging to them. Such debt obligations are hereby made securities which may properly and legally be deposited with and received by any commonwealth or municipal officer or any agency or political subdivision of the commonwealth for any purpose for which the deposit of bonds or obligations of the commonwealth is now or may hereafter be authorized by law.

(k) Debt obligations issued by the city under the provisions of this section shall not be deemed to be a debt or a pledge of the faith and credit of the city but shall be payable solely from the funds of the hospital from which they are made payable pursuant to the provisions of this section. All debt obligations issued by the city under the provisions of this section, their transfer and the income therefrom, including any profit made on the sale thereof shall at all times be free from taxation of every kind by the commonwealth and by the cities, towns and other political subdivisions in the commonwealth.

(l) Notwithstanding anything in this section to the contrary, the hospital shall be liable to the city in each year for an amount equal to the amount of principal and interest payments coming due in such year on outstanding bonds of the city issued for the purposes of the hospital, and the rights of the holders of any debt obligations issued under this section shall be subordinated to the right of the city to receive such amount.

Section 6H. In order to promote the hospital's ability to compete more effectively in the health care marketplace, and in furtherance of the other purposes of this act, notwithstanding sections 23A to 23C, inclusive, of chapter 39 of the General Laws applicable to meetings of the board of any of its committees, and section 10 of chapter 66 of the General Laws relating to the availability of public records as defined in clause Twenty-sixth of section 7 of chapter 4 of the General Laws, all writings and other records concerning the following shall not be deemed to be public records for the purposes of said section 6D, and executive sessions may be held concerning the following: rates and charges; contracts and other arrangements with health care purchasers or with health care systems, or a constituent or affiliate thereof, with which the hospital is affiliated or is proposing to affiliate, including contracts relating to clinical service arrangements; medical records; and marketing strategies, strategic plans or other plans, analyses, evaluations, data or programs, if disclosure is deemed by the board to be likely to give an unfair competitive or bargaining advantage to any person or entity. This section shall not be construed to modify the provisions of the statutes cited in this paragraph as they otherwise apply to records, meetings and deliberations of the city council affecting the hospital, except that meetings and deliberations of the city council relating to its taking actions with respect to the hospital entering into affiliation arrangements, as provided in subsection (*a*) of section 6F may be in executive session, and all writings and other records provided to the hospital or to the city council by a health care system with which affiliation is under consideration by the hospital and the city council shall not be deemed to be public records for purposes of said section 10. Notwithstanding the foregoing, the seventh paragraph of section 23B of chapter 39 of the General Laws, relating to the records of and votes taken in executive sessions, shall apply to the records of and votes taken in executive sessions held by the board or any of its committees, or of the city council, with regard to any of the subject matters identified in this section for which executive sessions may be held. This section shall not be deemed to prevent access by an agency of the commonwealth to records of the hospital to which it would otherwise be entitled under other provisions of general or special law.

Section 6

Chapter 604 of the acts of 1987 is hereby repealed.

Section 7

Chapter 101 of the acts of 1993 is hereby repealed.

Section 8

This act shall take effect upon its passage.

Approved August 10, 2000.

EMERGENCY HEALTH SERVICE ACT, NOVA SCOTIA CANADA

An Act Respecting the Provision of Ambulance Services and Emergency Health Services

Be it enacted by the Governor and Assembly as follows:

1. This Act may be cited as the *Emergency Health Services Act*.

2. In this Act,

(a) "ambulance services" means services providing for the transport and stabilisation of patients and the dispatching of ambulances, and includes air and ground emergency and non-emergency ambulance services;

(b) "communications centre" means a centre that provides communications services for ambulance services;

(c) "emergency ambulance services" means ambulance services provided in situations that are determined by a communications-centre dispatcher to constitute an emergency requiring an immediate response;

(d) "emergency health services" means the arrangement of personnel, facilities and equipment required for the effective, co-ordinated delivery of services provided by registered pre-hospital first responders and by registered paramedics and other health professionals pursuant to this Act and required in the prevention and management of medical, trauma and health conditions;

(e) "hospital" means a hospital as defined in the Hospitals Act;

(f) "inspector" means an inspector appointed for the purpose of this Act;

(g) "Minister" means the Minister of Health;

(h) "Register" means the Register established or designated pursuant to this Act;

(i) "registered paramedic" means a paramedic whose name is on the Register;

(j) "registered pre-hospital first responder" means a pre-hospital first responder whose name is on the Register.

3. The Minister has the general supervision and management of this Act.

4. The Minister may undertake any function related to ambulance services, emergency health services and communications-centre services that the Minister considers necessary or advisable and, in particular, has the authority to

(a) ensure the existence throughout the Province of emergency health services, ambulance services and communications-centre services;

(b) make available the services of appropriately trained persons on a continuous, continual or temporary basis to enhance existing health services in any part of the Province;

(c) purchase, lease, sell, transfer or dispose of ambulances, equipment, facilities or other items as necessary for the administration of this Act; and

(d) monitor, inspect and evaluate ambulance services, emergency health services and communications-centre services, including facilities, equipment and supplies, and investigate complaints respecting them.

5. (1) Subject to the regulations, the Minister may establish standards for the management, operation and use of ground and air ambulances providing emergency or non-emergency services, for emergency health services and for communications-centre services and for any equipment, supplies and facilities required to provide the services and ensure compliance with those standards and, in particular, establish standards respecting

(a) clinical care and medical oversight in the provision of ambulance services, emergency health services and communications-centre services;

(b) trauma care;

(c) technical operations;

(d) emergency and non-emergency ambulance communications and dispatch;

(e) safe operation of air and ground ambulances;

(f) medical first response;

(g) facilities housing emergency health services operations.

(2) The exercise by the Minister of the authority contained

in this Section is regulations within the meaning of the Regulations Act.

6. The Minister may enter into agreements for the purpose of this Act with any person to provide ambulance services, emergency health services or communications-centre services in all or part of the Province.

7. No person shall operate the business or undertaking of providing ambulance services except pursuant to an agreement with the Minister.

8. The Minister may assist hospitals, other health institutions and agencies, municipalities and other organisations and persons to provide emergency health services and to train personnel to provide services, and to enter into agreements or arrangements for that purpose.

9. The Minister may establish one or more communications centres for the dispatch of ambulances throughout the Province.

10. Inspectors required for the purpose of this Act shall be appointed by the Minister.

11. (1) An inspector may, at any reasonable time, enter and inspect facilities used for the purpose of providing ambulance services, emergency health services, communications-centre services, the vehicles used for the provision of emergency and non-emergency ambulance services, and any other equipment and supplies used in the provision of ambulance services, emergency health services and communications-centre services.

(2) Any person who is operating an ambulance service, providing an emergency health service or operating a communications centre shall permit an inspector, at any reasonable time, to enter and inspect the facility used for

the provision of ambulance services, emergency health services, communications-centre services, the vehicles used in the provision of emergency and non-emergency ambulance services, and all equipment and supplies.

(3) Any person providing ambulance services, emergency health services or communications-centre services shall forward to an inspector such records, returns, and reports as the inspector requests, in the form and manner and within the time the inspector requests.

12. Where there are reasonable grounds to believe that an ambulance is being operated in violation of this Act or the regulations, an inspector may detain the ambulance in accordance with policies established by the Minister.

13. No ambulance shall be used for purposes other than ambulance transport, public education or other activities authorized by the Minister.

14. The Minister shall

(a) establish a Register of pre-hospital first responders, paramedics and emergency medical dispatchers; or

(b) designate a register maintained by a regulatory body with authority to register paramedics and emergency medical dispatchers.

15. No paramedic or emergency medical dispatcher whose name is not on the Register shall be employed as a paramedic or emergency medical dispatcher under this Act.

16. A paramedic or emergency medical dispatcher employed under this Act shall work in accordance with patient-care standards and procedures established pursuant to this Act.

17. (1) Every person who contravenes or fails to comply

with this Act or the regulations is liable on summary conviction to a penalty of not more than ten thousand dollars.

(2) Every day on which an offence continues constitutes a separate offence.

18. (1) The Governor in Council may make regulations

(a) respecting clinical care and safety of pre-hospital patients receiving ambulance services and emergency health services;

(b) respecting the operation of ambulance services;

(c) respecting performance standards and monitoring and enforcement of those standards;

(d) respecting educational and other programs to provide up-to-date pre-hospital health services;

(e) prescribing data to be collected respecting ambulance services and emergency health services;

(f) prescribing standards for the design, structure and licensing of ambulances;

(g) respecting the equipment, medication and supplies that must be carried in an ambulance;

(h) respecting the maintenance, repair and inspection of ambulances and the equipment used in ambulances;

(i) respecting any matter necessary or advisable for the acceptance of bequests, grants and donations and for the undertaking of fundraising events to support the provision of ambulance services;

(j) respecting the development of programs using the communications centre;

(k) defining any word or expression used but not defined in this Act;

(l) respecting any matter that the Governor in Council considers necessary or advisable to carry out effectively the intent and purpose of this Act.

(2) The exercise by the Governor in Council of the authority contained in this Section is regulations within the meaning of the Regulations Act.

19. Chapter 8 of the Acts of 1994, the Emergency Health Services Agency Act, is repealed.

20. This Act comes into force on such day as the Governor in Council orders and declares by proclamation.

3

Regulations for Hospital and Diagnostic Centres

1. In this Act

"authorized charges" Repealed: 1986, c.43, s.1.

"cost of th e entitled services" includes the cost of future entitled services;

"entitled services" means the insured hospital and diagnostic services to which a person is entitled under this Act and the regulations without charge, if received in the Province, and in accordance with the rates established under the hospital services plan, if received outside the Province;

"fiscal year" means the period commencing on April 1 in one year and ending on March 31 in the next year;

"hospital" Repealed: 1992, c.52, s.16.

"hospital corporation" Repealed: 2002, c.1, s.12.

"medical practitioner" means a member of the medical profession who is licensed to practise medicine under the laws of the jurisdiction in which the medical practitioner practises;

"Minister" means the Minister of Health and includes any person designated by the Minister to act on his or her behalf;

"oral and maxillofacial surgeon" means a dental practitioner whose name is entered in the specialists register and who is the holder of a specialist's licence in oral and maxillofacial surgery issued pursuant to the *New Brunswick Dental Act, 1985*, or a dental practitioner who practises outside of New Brunswick and who is recognized as an oral and maxillofacial surgeon by the licensing body of the jurisdiction in which that dental practitioner practises oral and maxillofacial surgery;

"regional health authority" means a regional health authority as defined in the *Regional Health Authorities Act*;

"resident" or "resident of the Province" means a resident as defined in the regulations.

1960-61, c.11, s.1; 1979, c.33, s.1; 1983, c.38, s.1; 1986, c.8, s.56; 1986, c.43, s.1; 1992, c.52, s.16; 1992, c.81, s.1; 1993, c.61, s.1; 1997, c.18, s.1; 2000, c.26, s.159; 2002, c.1, s.12; 2003, c.21, s.1; 2006, c.16, s.85.

2. The Government of New Brunswick, represented by the Minister of Health, may enter into and amend from time to time an agreement with the Government of Canada under which Canada will contribute to the cost of entitled services provided for in this Act in accordance with such terms and conditions as the agreement may provide.

1960-61, c.11, s.2; 1986, c.8, s.56; 2000, c.26, s.159; 2006, c.16, s.85.

3. The Minister shall administer and enforce this Act and the regulations and may designate another person to act on his behalf.

1960-61, c.11, s.3; 1979, c.33, s.2.

4. The Minister may take such steps as he deems necessary for the following purposes:

(a) to ensure the development throughout New Brunswick of a balanced and integrated system of hospital facilities,

(b) to approve regional health authorities for the purposes of this Act in accordance with the regulations,

(b.1) to approve hospitals and other facilities outside New Brunswick for the purposes of this Act in accordance with the regulations,

(c) to approve the establishment of new hospital facilities and additions to existing hospital facilities,

(d) to determine the amount of and pay for hospital facility construction,

(e) Repealed: 2002, c.1, s.12.

(f) Repealed: 2002, c.1, s.12.

(g) to administer the hospital services plan established by the regulations,

(h) to determine the amounts to be paid to regional health authorities and to pay regional health authorities for entitled services provided to persons under the hospital services plan and to make retroactive adjustments with regional health authorities for underpayment and overpayment for entitled services according to the cost as determined in accordance with this Act and the regulations,

(h.1) to determine the amounts to be paid and to pay for entitled services received or to be received by entitled persons under the hospital services plan from hospitals and other facilities outside New Brunswick and to make retroactive adjustments for underpayment and overpayment for such entitled services according to the cost as determined in accordance with this Act and the regulations,

(h.2) to determine the amounts to be paid to and to pay hospitals and other facilities outside New Brunswick for services provided under the hospital services plan and to make retroactive adjustments with those hospitals and other facilities for underpayment and overpayment for services according to the cost as determined in accordance with this Act and the regulations,

(i) to control all charges made to patients by regional health authorities in New Brunswick to which payments are made under the hospital services plan,

(j) to prescribe forms necessary or desirable to carry out the intent and purposes of this Act and the regulations,

(k) to appoint medical practitioners, oral and maxillofacial surgeons and other health professionals with the duty and power to examine and obtain information from the clinical and other regional health authority records, reports and accounts of patients who are receiving or who have received entitled services,

(k.1) to appoint medical practitioners, oral and maxillofacial surgeons and other health professionals with the duty and power to examine and obtain information from the clinical and other records, reports and accounts of patients who are receiving or who have received entitled services from hospitals and other facilities outside New Brunswick,

(l) Repealed: 2002, c.1, s.12.

(l.1) to appoint inspectors and other officers with the duty and power to examine and obtain information from the accounting records, books, returns, reports and audited financial statements and reports thereon of hospitals and other facilities outside New Brunswick to which payments are made directly or indirectly under the hospital services plan,

(m) to withhold payment for entitled services in respect of any person who does not, in the opinion of the Minister, medically require such services,

(n) to enter into agreements with hospitals and other facilities outside New Brunswick, and with other governments and with hospital service authorities established by other governments, for providing services under the hospital services plan, and

(o) to perform such other functions and discharge such other duties as may be prescribed from time to time by the Lieutenant-Governor in Council.

1960-61, c.11, s.4; 1967, c.47, s.1; 1992, c.52, s.16; 1992, c.78, s.1; 2002, c.1, s.12; 2003, c.21, s.2.

4.01. (1) In this section

"target fiscal year" means the 2000-2001 fiscal year unless the Lieutenant-Governor in Council prescribes another fiscal year to be the target fiscal year.

4.01. (2) Where, on or after July 1, 1993, a regional health authority grants privileges to a medical practitioner who becomes engaged in a type of practice in an area of the Province during a fiscal year and the effect of that medical practitioner engaging in that type of practice in that area is to, at the time the medical practitioner becomes so engaged,

(a) cause the actual number of full time equivalents for that type of practice in that area in the fiscal year to exceed the maximum desirable level of full time equivalents established by the provincial authority for that type of practice in that area for the fiscal year or for the target fiscal year, as determined in accordance with the Medical Services Payment Act and regulations,

(b) increase the actual number of full time equivalents for that type of practice in that area in the fiscal year where the actual number of full time equivalents exceeds the maximum desirable level of full time equivalents established by the provincial authority for that type of practice in that area for the fiscal year or for the target fiscal year, as determined in accordance with the Medical Services Payment Act and regulations, or

(c) fail to reduce the actual number of full time equivalents for that type of practice in that area in the fiscal year where the actual number of full time equivalents exceeds the maximum desirable level of full time equivalents established by the provincial authority for that type of practice in that area for the target fiscal year, as determined in accordance with the *Medical Services Payment Act* and regulations,

the Minister may withhold money, in accordance with a formula provided in the regulations, from the operating budget of the regional health authority who grants the privileges.

4.01(3) The Minister may transfer the money withheld under this section to the operating budget of the medical services plan established under the *Medical Services Payment Act*.

4.01(4) Where subsection (3) conflicts with a provision in any other Act, subsection (3) prevails.

4.01(5) Notwithstanding section 8 of the *Medical Services Payment Act*, information with respect to payments by Medicare to a medical practitioner who has an effect described in paragraph (2)(a), (b) or (c) shall be communicated to the Minister for the purposes of withholding money under this section.

1993, c.61, s.2; 2002, c.1, s.12.

4.1 Repealed: 1986, c.43, s.2.

1979, c.33, s.2.1; 1983, c.38, s.2; 1986, c.43, s.2.

5 Neither Her Majesty the Queen in right of the Province nor the Minister is liable for any act or omission of any regional health authority official, any person on the medical staff or nursing staff of a regional health authority or any employee or agent of a regional health authority.

1960-61, c.11, s.5; 1992, c.52, s.16; 1992, c.78, s.2; 2003, c.21, s.3.

5.1 Neither Her Majesty the Queen in right of the Province nor the Minister is liable for any act or omission of an official, a member of the medical staff or nursing staff, or an employee or agent of a hospital or other facility outside New Brunswick to which payments are made directly or indirectly under the hospital services plan.

1992, c.78, s.3.

5.2 No action for damages or other proceeding shall be taken against any committee established under this Act or the regulations or the *Medical Services Payment Act* or the regulations under that Act, or any member of such committee, with respect to anything done or purported to be done in good faith by the committee or as a member of such committee, or with respect to anything omitted to be done in good faith by the committee or as a member of such committee, under this Act or the regulations.

1998, c.10, s.1.

6(1) No person shall knowingly obtain or receive entitled services that he is not entitled to obtain or receive under this Act and the regulations.

6(2) No person shall knowingly aid or abet another person to obtain or receive entitled services that such other person is not entitled to obtain or receive under this Act and the regulations.

6(3) A person who violates or fails to comply with subsection (1) or (2) commits an offence punishable under Part II of the *Provincial Offences Procedure Act* as a category F offence.

1960-61, c.11, s.6; 1990, c.61, s.63.

7 A person who obstructs an inspector or other officer who is acting pursuant to this Act and the regulations commits an offence punishable under Part II of the *Provincial Offences Procedure Act* as a category E offence.

1960-61, c.11, s.7; 1990, c.61, s.63.

8 A person who violates or fails to comply with any provision of the regulations commits an offence punishable under Part II of the *Provincial Offences Procedure Act* as a category B offence.

1960-61, c.11, s.8; 1990, c.61, s.63.

9(1) The Lieutenant-Governor in Council may make such regulations as may be deemed necessary for the following purposes:

(a) establishing a hospital services plan;

(b) making entitled services available to all residents of the Province upon uniform terms and conditions;

(b.1) prescribing a target fiscal year;

(b.2) respecting formulas for the withholding of money from the operating budget of a regional health authority under section 4.01;

(c) approving regional health authorities for the purposes of the hospital services plan;

(c.1) approving hospitals and other facilities outside New Brunswick for the purposes of the hospital services plan;

(d) making such arrangements as are necessary to ensure that adequate standards are maintained in hospital facilities established, operated and maintained, or operated and maintained by regional health authorities;

(d.1) making such arrangements as are necessary to ensure that adequate standards are maintained in hospitals and other facilities outside New Brunswick to which payments are made directly or indirectly under the hospital services plan;

(e) providing for the admission, discipline and discharge of patients or any class of patients of regional health authorities in New Brunswick to which payments are made under the hospital services plan;

(e.01) providing for the admission, discipline and discharge of patients or any class of patients in hospitals or other facilities outside New Brunswick to which payments are made directly or indirectly under the hospital services plan;

(e.1) respecting the payment of a fee to a barrister and solicitor who makes a claim on behalf of an injured person and recovers a sum in respect of the cost of entitled services in accordance with section 10;

(f) regulating the making and renewing of contracts of insurance and pre-payment plans with residents to provide any benefits related directly or indirectly to hospitalization or to the length of time a person is hospitalized;

(g) Repealed: 1988, c.18, s.1.

(g.1) prescribing the terms and conditions under which Her Majesty and a person who has suffered personal injuries as a result of the negligence or wrongful act of another shall share the proceeds of any recovery under subsection 10(7);

(h) defining words used in the Act for the purposes of this Act and the regulations;

(h.1) Repealed: 1986, c.43, s.3.

(i) respecting any other matter necessary or advisable to carry out effectively the intent and purposes of this Act.

9(2) Any regulation may be limited in its application in time, place, persons or things, and subject to the agreement under section 2, may be retroactive in its operation.

1960-61, c.11, s.9; 1979, c.33, s.3; 1985, c.13, s.1; 1986, c.43, s.3; 1988, c.18, s.1; 1992, c.52, s.16; 1992, c.78, s.4; 1993, c.61, s.3; 2002, c.1, s.12; 2003, c.21, s.4.

10(1) Where, as a result of the negligence or wrongful act of another, a person suffers personal injuries for which he receives entitled services under this Act or the regulations, he

(a) shall have the same right to claim and to recover the cost of the entitled services against the person who was negligent or who did the wrongful act as he would have had if he, himself, had been required to pay for the entitled services, and

(b) if he makes any claim for the personal injuries suffered against the person who was negligent or who did the wrongful act, shall claim and seek to recover the cost of the entitled services.

10(2) Where under subsection (1), a person either acting for himself or on behalf of another person, recovers a sum in respect of entitled services received under this Act or the regulations, he shall as soon as practicable pay such sum recovered to the Minister.

10(3) Where, as a result of the negligence or wrongful act of another, a person suffers personal injuries for which he receives entitled services under this Act or the regulations and he does not claim against the person who was negligent or who did the wrongful act, Her Majesty the Queen in right of the Province may maintain an action in her own name or in the name of the injured person for recovery of the cost of the entitled services.

10(4) Where, as a result of the negligence or wrongful act of another, a person suffers personal injuries for which he receives entitled services under this Act or the regulations and a claim is made against the person who was negligent or who did the wrongful act but the person making the claim, either acting on his own behalf or on behalf of another person, does not

(a) claim for the cost of the entitled services,

(b) if a release is given or the claim is settled, obtain a written approval of the release or settlement in accordance with subsection (9) or (10), or

(c) pay any sum recovered in respect of the entitled services to the Minister in accordance with subsection (2),

Her Majesty the Queen in Right of the Province may maintain an action in her own name against the person making the claim, whether acting on his own behalf or on behalf of another person, for recovery of the cost of the entitled services.

10(5) It shall not be a defence to an action brought by Her Majesty under subsection (4) that a release has been given, a claim has been settled or a judgment obtained unless

(a) the claim included a claim for the cost of the entitled services, and

(b) if a release is given or the claim is settled, the Minister has under subsection (9) or (10) approved the release or settlement.

10(6) Where the Minister approves in writing a release or settlement under subsection (10), Her Majesty the Queen in right of the Province may continue the action or maintain an action in her own name for recovery of the cost of the entitled services.

10(7) Subject to subsection (10), where, as a result of a claim under this section

(a) the claim is settled or a judgment is obtained, and

(b) insufficient funds are available to provide complete

recovery to the injured person for his losses and injuries and to pay the cost of the entitled services, the injured person and Her Majesty the Queen in right of the Province shall share *pro rata* in proportion to their respective losses in any recovery in accordance with the terms and conditions prescribed by regulation.

10(8) No person, acting for himself or on behalf of another person, shall, without the approval in writing under subsection (9) or (10) of the Minister make a settlement of a claim based upon a cause of action for damages for personal injuries in a case where the injured person has received entitled services under this Act or the regulations unless at the same time he makes a settlement to recover the same *pro rata* proportion in respect of the cost of the entitled services as the injured person is to recover in respect of his losses and injuries.

10(9) No release or settlement of a claim or judgment based upon a cause of action for damages for personal injuries in a case where the injured person has received entitled services under this Act or the regulations is binding upon Her Majesty unless the Minister has approved the release or settlement in writing.

10(10) Notwithstanding subsection (9), where a person who makes a claim under subsection (1) has obtained an offer for a settlement whereby the same *pro rata* proportion of the cost of entitled services would be recovered as the injured person would recover in respect of his losses and injuries but, in the opinion of the Minister, the offer would not provide sufficient recovery in respect of the entitled services, the Minister may approve in writing a release or settlement whereby the person making a claim under subsection (1) makes a settlement of a claim in respect of his injuries or losses without making a settlement in respect of the cost of the entitled services but the written approval is not binding on Her Majesty in relation to a claim made under subsection (6) in respect of the cost of the entitled services.

10(11) Where a person whose negligent or wrongful act resulted in personal injuries to another is insured by a liability insurer carrying on business in the Province and a claim made in respect of those personal injuries does not include a claim for the cost of the entitled services received by the injured person under this Act or the regulations, the liability insurer shall pay to the Minister the cost of the entitled services and payment of that amount to the Minister discharges the liability of the insurer to pay the cost of the entitled services in any subsequent claim to the insured person or any person claiming under or on behalf of the insured person.

10(12) Every liability insurer carrying on business in the Province shall provide the Minister, when requested to do so, information relating to

(a) a claim made against an insured person by a person who received entitled services under this Act or the regulations, or

(b) the terms and conditions of any settlement entered into by an insured person and a person who received entitled services under this Act or the regulations.

10(13) In an action under this section a certificate signed or purporting to be signed by or on behalf of the Minister shall be accepted by all courts

(a) as conclusive proof

(i) that the person named in the certificate has received entitled services,

(ii) that the amount recorded in the certificate is the cost of the entitled services received by the person named in the certificate, and

(iii) of the office, authority and signature of the person signing or purporting to sign the certificate, without proof of his appointment, authority or signature, and

(b) as prima facie proof that the entitled services were received in respect of the personal injuries suffered.

10(14) This section applies except where the personal injuries occurred as a result of the use or operation of a motor vehicle registered in the Province.

10.01 The Minister may, in accordance with the *Insurance Act*, impose a levy for the purpose of recovering the cost of the entitled services provided to persons under this Act as a result of personal injuries arising out of the use or operation of a motor vehicle registered in the Province.

10.1 Notwithstanding any other provision of this Act, the Minister may, in accordance with the regulations, authorize the payment of a fee to a barrister and solicitor who makes a claim on behalf of an injured person and recovers a sum in respect of the cost of entitled services in accordance with section 10.

11 In the event of conflict between any provision of this Act and any provision of any other Act of New Brunswick, the provision of this Act prevails.

N.B. This Act is consolidated to June 22, 2006.

4

Guidelines for Nursing Home and Medical Devices Administration

REGULATIONS FOR THE SUPERVISION AND ADMINISTRATION OF MEDICAL DEVICES IN CHINBA

(Entry into Force: April 2000)

I. GENERAL PROVISIONS

Article 1

These Regulations are hereby formulated with a view to strengthening the supervision and administration of medical devices, ensuring their safety and effectiveness and protecting human health and life safety.

Article 2

All units or individuals engaged in the research and development, production, distribution, use, supervision and administration of medical devices within the territory of the People's Republic of China shall comply with the Regulation.

Article 3

"Medical devices" as defined by these regulations refers to: any instrument, apparatus, appliance, material, or other article whether used alone or in combination, including the software necessary for its proper application. It does not achieve its principal action in or on the human body by means of pharmacology, immunology or metabolism, but which may be assisted in its function by such means; the use of which is to achieve the following intended objectives:

1. Diagnosis, prevention, monitoring, treatment or alleviation of disease;
2. Diagnosis, monitoring, treatment, alleviation of or compensation for an injury or handicap conditions;
3. Investigation, replacement or modification for anatomy or a physiological process;
4. Control of conception.

Article 4

The drug regulatory authority under the State Council is responsible for supervision and administration of medical devices nationwide. The drug administration of the local government at county level and above is responsible for supervision and administration of medical devices in each administrative region. The drug regulatory authority under the State Council shall coordinate with other departments under the State Council, responsible for comprehensive economic administration, in the implementation of policies for the medical device industry.

Article 5

The State shall classify medical devices and administer them based on this classification

Class I Medical Devices are those for which safety and effectiveness can be ensured through routine administration;

Class II Medical Devices are those for which further control is required to ensure their safety and effectiveness

Class III Medical Devices are those which are implanted into the human body, or used for life support or sustenance, or pose potential risk to the human body and thus must be strictly controlled in respect to safety and effectiveness.

The classification catalogue for medical devices shall be stipulated, adjusted and promulgated by the drug regulatory authority under the State Council, in accordance with classification principles after consulting with health authority under the State Council.

Article 6

Medical devices produced and used for the purpose of providing concrete measuring values shall comply with the requirements of the metering law. The detailed product list shall be formulated and promulgated by the drug regulatory authority under the State Council, jointly with the metering authority.

II. THE ADMINISTRATION OF MEDICAL DEVICES

Article 7

The State encourages the research and development of new medical devices. "New medical devices" refer to the kind of brand new product varieties which have not been available in the domestic market, or for which the safety, effectiveness and product mechanism have not been recognized domestically.

The clinical trials of new medical devices of Class II and Class III can be conducted only after clinical trial approval by the relevant authority in accordance with the rules of the drug regulatory authority under State Council.

New medical devices that have completed clinical trials and passed experts' evaluation and review organised by the drug regulatory authority under State Council, shall receive a new product certificate after being approved by the same organisation.

Article 8

The State shall implement a product registration system for the manufacturing of medical devices.

Class I medical devices shall be inspected, approved and granted with a registration certificate by the drug regulatory authority of the government of the municipalities consisting of districts.

Class II medical devices shall be inspected, approved and granted with registration certificates by the drug regulatory authorities of provinces, autonomous regions and municipalities directly under the central government.

Class III medical devices shall be inspected, approved and granted with registration certificates by the drug regulatory authority directly under the State Council.

Clinical evaluation must be conducted for Class II and Class III medical devices before they are put into production.

Article 9

The drug regulatory authorities of provinces, autonomous regions and municipalities directly under the central government are responsible for the inspection and approval of the clinical trial or verification of class II medical devices in their own administrative regions. The drug regulatory authority under the State Council is responsible for the inspection and approval of clinical trial or verification of class III medical devices.

Clinical trial or verification shall be conducted in the medical institutions designated by the drug regulatory authorities of the government at provincial level and above. The medical institutions shall conduct the clinical trial or verification, in accordance with the related provisions of the drug regulatory authority under the State Council.

The qualification of medical institutions engaged in the clinical trial or verification shall be certified by the drug regulatory authority, jointly with the health authority under the State Council.

Article 10

Medical institutions may develop medical devices to serve their own clinical needs, and use them within their own institution under the guidance of licensed medical practitioners.

Class II medical devices developed by medical institutions shall be inspected and approved by the drug regulatory authority of the government at provincial level and above. Class III medical devices developed by medical institutions shall be inspected and approved by the drug regulatory authority under the State Council.

Article 11

When importing medical devices into China for the first time, the agent of the imported device, should submit the instruction for use, quality standards, testing methods, other relevant information, product samples, and marketing authorisation certificates issued by the manufacturing countries (regions), for inspection and approval by the drug regulatory authority under the State Council, and receive an import product registration certificate before applying for customs formalities.

Article 12

When applying for registration of medical devices, technical standards, testing report and other relevant information shall be submitted according to provisions of the drug regulatory authority under the State Council.

The drug regulatory authority of the government of the

municipality consisting of districts shall decide within 30 working days if the product can be registered, counting from the date of acceptance of the application. For those not approved for registration, a written explanation shall be given to the applicant.

The drug regulatory authority of governments of provinces, autonomous regions and municipalities directly under central government shall decide within 60 working days if the product can be registered, counting from the date of acceptance of the application. For those not approved for registration, a written explanation shall be given to the applicant.

The drug regulatory authority under the State Council shall decide within 90 working days if the product can be registered, counting from the date of acceptance of the application. For those not approved for registration, a written explanation shall be given to the applicant.

Article 13

In case any situation reflected in the content of the registration certificate is changed, the holder of the certificate shall apply for an amendment of the certificate accordingly, or for re-registration within 30 working days from the change.

Article 14

The term of validity for the registration certificate of medical devices is four years. The holder of the certificate shall apply for re-registration within six months before the certificate expires.

When the manufacturing of a medical device is stopped continuously for more than 2 years, its registration certificate is automatically invalidated.

Article 15

Medical devices manufactured shall meet the national standard, or professional standards when there are no relevant national standards available.

National standards of medical devices shall be formulated jointly by the standardisation authority and the drug regulatory authority under the State Council. Professional standards of medical devices shall be formulated by the drug regulatory authority under the State Council.

Article 16

The instruction for use, label and package of medical devices shall comply with relevant standards or provisions in China.

Article 17

The registration number of a medical device shall be marked on the product itself and the external package according to the provisions of the drug regulatory authority under the State Council.

Article 18

The State implements a system of re-evaluation and obsolescence for medical devices, the details of which shall be formulated by drug regulatory authority under the State Council after consulting with other related authorities under the State Council.

III. ADMINISTRATION OF PRODUCTION, DISTRIBUTION AND USE OF MEDICAL DEVICES

Article 19

Enterprises manufacturing medical devices shall meet the following conditions:

1. Possess professional technical personnel required for the manufacture of its medical devices;
2. Possess facility and environment required for the manufacture of its medical devices;
3. Possess equipment required for the manufacture of its medical devices;
4. Possess an establishment or personnel and equipment for quality testing required for the manufacture of its medical devices.

Article 20

Establishment of manufacturing of class I medical devices, requires that the enterprise file a record with the drug regulatory authority of provinces, autonomous regions or municipalities directly under the central government.

Establishing manufacturing of class II and/or class III medical devices, requires inspection and approval by the drug regulatory authorities of the provinces, autonomous regions and municipalities directly under the central government, who will then issue a Medical Device Manufacturing Enterprise License. The industrial and commercial authority shall not issue a business license to enterprises which have not received a Medical Device Manufacturing Enterprise License.

The term of validity of the Medical Device Manufacturing Enterprise License is 5 years. Upon expiration, re-inspection and license renewal shall be conducted. Implementation details shall be formulated by the drug regulatory authority under the State Council.

Article 21

Medical device manufacturing enterprises shall not start manufacturing products before obtaining the manufacturing enterprise license.

Article 22

The State implements a mandatory safety certification system for certain class III medical devices. A specific product list shall be established by the drug regulatory authority under the State Council, jointly with the quality and technology supervision authority.

Article 23

Enterprises distributing medical devices shall meet the following conditions:

1. Possess appropriate facility(s) and environment for the kind of medical devices to be distributed;
2. Possess appropriate quality inspection personnel for the kind of medical devices to be distributed;
3. Possess adequate ability for technical training, maintenance and after-sales services for the kinds of medical devices to be distributed;

Article 24

Establishing of distribution of class II and/or class III medical devices, requires that the enterprise file a record with the drug regulatory authority of provinces, autonomous regions or municipalities directly under the central government.

Establishing an enterprise distributing class II and/or class III medical devices, requires inspection and approval by the drug regulatory authorities of the provinces, autonomous regions and municipalities directly under the central government, who will then issue a Medical Device Distributing Enterprise License. The industrial and commercial authority shall not issue a business license to enterprises which have not received a Medical Device Distributing Enterprise License.

The term of validity of the Medical Device Distribution Enterprise License is 5 years. Upon expiration, re-inspection and license renewal shall be conducted. Implementation details shall be formulated by the drug regulatory authority under the State Council.

Article 25

The drug regulatory authority of governments of provinces, autonomous regions and municipalities directly under central government shall decide within 30 working days whether the licenses for manufacturing or distributing enterprises of medical devices can be issued, counting from the date of acceptance of the application. When a license is not issued, a written explanation shall be given to the applicant.

Article 26

Distribution enterprises and medical institutions shall purchase qualified medical devices from enterprises having a Medical Device Manufacturing Enterprise License or Medical Device Distribution Enterprise License, and shall verify the certificates of qualified products.

Distribution enterprises shall not distribute medical devices without registration certificates or certificates for qualified products, or medical devices which are beyond their expiry dates, of compromised effectiveness, or obsolete.

Medical institutions shall not use medical devices without registration, or certificate for qualified products, or medical devices which are beyond their expiry dates, of compromised effectiveness, or obsolete.

Article 27

Medical institutions shall not re-use medical devices labeled for single use, shall destroy them after use and establish a record, according to relevant provisions of the country.

Article 28

The State shall establish a quality incident reporting system and a warning system of medical devices. Implementation details shall be stipulated by the drug regulatory authority under the State Council, in conjunction with the health authority and family planning authority under the State Council.

IV. SUPERVISION OF MEDICAL DEVICES

Article 29

The drug regulatory authorities of governments at county level and above shall appoint medical device monitors within their organisation, who are responsible for the supervision and inspection of medical device manufacturing enterprises, distribution enterprises and medical institutions within their own administrative regions. When necessary, monitors may take product samples and ask for relevant materials according to the provisions promulgated by the drug regulatory authority under the State Council. Institutions and individuals concerned shall not decline cooperation or be deceitful in the monitoring process. The monitors shall be responsible to keep collected samples and materials confidential.

Article 30

The State implements an accreditation system for the qualification of the testing institutions of medical devices. Only testing institutions accredited by the drug regulatory authority in conjunction with the quality and technical supervision authority under the State Council may conduct medical device test.

Medical device testing institutions and their staff members shall keep strictly confidential all technical information provided by enterprises whose products are being tested, and shall not conduct or be involved in research and development, manufacture, distribution and technical consultation related to the devices tested.

Article 31

For products having caused or which may potentially cause quality incidents, the drug regulatory authority of the governments at county level and above shall have the right to check, seal up and detain them together with materials related.

Article 32

The drug regulatory authority of the governments at provincial level and above shall revoke the registration certificates of medical devices of which safety and effectiveness can not be ensured. Medical devices whose registration certificates have been revoked shall not be manufactured, distributed and used. Those already produced or imported shall be dealt with by the drug regulatory authority of government at county level and above.

Article 33

The drug regulatory authorities of the government of the municipality consisting of districts and above, which perform product registrations in violation of these regulations, shall be ordered by the drug regulatory authority under the state council to correct the violations within a defined period. For those not corrected within the period, the product registration certificates may be revoked and the events may be made public.

Article 34

Advertisements of medical devices shall be reviewed

and approved by the drug regulatory authority of governments at provincial level and above, and shall not be published, broadcasted, circulated or posted before the approval.

The contents of the advertisements shall be based on the instruction for use approved by the drug regulatory authority under the State Council or the drug regulatory authority of the governments of provinces, autonomous regions and municipalities directly under the Central Government.

V. PENALTIES

Article 35

In cases of manufacturing medical devices without product registration certificates, in violation of provisions of these Regulations, the drug regulatory authority of governments at county level and above shall issue an order to stop the production, confiscate all of the illegally manufactured products and related illegal income. Additionally, in case the illegal incomes exceed RMB10 thousand yuan, a fine of 3 to 5 times the total sum of the illegal income shall be imposed; in case there are no illegal incomes or the illegal incomes do not exceed RMB10 thousand yuan, a fine of RMB10 thousand yuan to RMB30 thousand yuan shall be imposed; in serious cases, the drug regulatory authorities of the governments at the provinces, autonomous regions and municipalities directly under the Central Government shall revoke the Medical Device Manufacturing Enterprise License; and in case crimes are committed, criminal liability shall be investigated and handled according to the law.

Article 36

In cases of manufacturing class II and class III medical devices without a Medical Device Manufacturing Enterprise

License, in violation of these regulations, the drug regulatory authority of governments at county level and above shall issue an order to stop the production, confiscate all of the illegally manufactured products and their illegal incomes. Additionally, in case the illegal incomes exceed RMB10 thousand yuan, a fine of 3 to 5 times of the total sum of the illegal incomes shall be imposed; in case there are no illegal incomes or the illegal incomes do not exceed RMB10 thousand yuan, a fine of RMB10 thousand yuan to RMB30 thousand yuan shall be imposed; and in case crimes are committed, criminal liability shall be investigated and handled according to the law.

Article 37

In cases of manufacturing medical devices not in conformity with national standards or professional standards for medical devices, in violation of provisions of these Regulations, the drug regulatory authority of governments at county level and above shall issue an warning, followed with an order to stop the production, confiscate all of the illegally manufactured products and their illegal incomes. Additionally, in case the illegal incomes exceed RMB 5 thousand yuan, a fine of 2 to 5 times of the total sum of the illegal incomes shall be imposed; in case there are no illegal incomes or the illegal incomes do not exceed RMB 5 thousand yuan, a fine of RMB 5 thousand to 20 thousand yuan shall be imposed; in serious cases, the product registration certificates shall be revoked by the authorities originally issued the certificates; and in case crimes are committed, criminal liability shall be investigated and handled according to the law.

Article 38

In cases of Distribution of class II and class III medical devices without a Medical Device Distributing Enterprise

License, which violates provisions of these Regulations, the drug regulatory authority of governments at county level and above shall issue an order to stop the production, confiscate all of the illegally manufactured products and their illegal incomes. Additionally, in case the illegal incomes exceed RMB 5 thousand yuan, a fine of 2 to 5 times of the total sum of the illegal incomes shall be imposed; in case there are no illegal incomes or the illegal incomes do not exceed RMB 5 thousand yuan, a fine of RMB 5 thousand yuan to RMB 20 thousand yuan shall be imposed; and in case crimes are committed, criminal liability shall be investigated and handled according to the law.

Article 39

In cases of distributing medical devices without registration certificates or certificate for qualified products, or medical devices which are beyond their expiry dates, of compromised effectiveness, or obsolete, or purchasing medical devices from enterprises without Medical Device Manufacturing Enterprise License or Medical Device Distributing Enterprise License, which violates provisions of these Regulations, the drug regulatory authority of governments at county level and above shall issue an order to stop the distribution, confiscate all of the illegally distributed products and their illegal incomes. Additionally, in case the illegal incomes exceed RMB 5 thousand yuan, a fine of 2 to 5 times of the total sum of the illegal incomes shall be imposed; in case there are no illegal incomes or the illegal incomes do not exceed RMB 5 thousand yuan, a fine of RMB 5 thousand to 20 thousand yuan shall be imposed; in serious cases, the Medical Device Distributing Enterprise License shall be revoked by the authorities which originally issued the license; and in case crimes are committed, criminal liability shall be investigated and handled according to the law.

Article 40

In cases where false certificates, documents, materials, or product samples are submitted in registration applications, or obtaining medical device registration certificates are obtained using other deceitful means, which violate provisions of these Regulations, the product registration certificates shall be revoked by the authorities which originally issued the certificates, and within a period of two years, other product registration applications of the violating enterprise shall not be accepted. Additionally, a fine of RMB 10 thousand to 30 thousand yuan shall be imposed; for enterprises already started manufacturing, all of the illegally manufactured products and their illegal incomes shall be confiscated; in case the illegal incomes exceed RMB10 thousand yuan, a fine of 3 to 5 times of the total sum of the illegal incomes shall be imposed; in case there are no illegal incomes or the illegal incomes do not exceed RMB10 thousand yuan, a fine of RMB 10 thousand to 30 thousand yuan shall be imposed; and in case crimes are committed, criminal liability shall be investigated and handled according to the law.

Article 41

Violation of Article 34 of these Regulations concerning provisions for advertisement of medical devices shall be dealt with by the industrial and commercial authority according to relevant laws and regulations of the country.

Article 42

In cases of Medical institutions using medical devices without registration certificates or certificate for qualified products, or medical devices which are beyond their expiry dates, of compromised effectiveness, or obsolete, or purchasing medical devices from enterprises without Medical Device Manufacturing Enterprise License or Medical Device Distributing Enterprise License, which violate provisions of these Regulations, the drug regulatory authority of governments at county level and above shall issue an order for correction, launch a warning, and confiscate all of the illegally used products and illegal incomes. Additionally, in case the illegal incomes exceed RMB 5 thousand yuan, a fine of 2 tb 5 times of the total sum of the illegal incomes shall be imposed; in case there are no illegal incomes or the illegal incomes do not exceed RMB 5 thousand yuan, a fine of RMB 5 thousand to 20 thousand yuan shall be imposed, and person(s) in charge and other directly responsible personnel shall receive disciplinary punishment; and in case crimes are committed, criminal liability shall be investigated and handled according to the law.

Article 43

In cases of medical institutions re-using devices for single use, or not destroying devices which should be destroyed, which violates provisions of these Regulations, the drug regulatory authority of governments at county level and above shall issue an order for correction and launch a warning, and may impose a fine of RMB 5 thousand to 30 thousand yuan; in serious cases, the medical institutions may be applied with a fine of RMB 30 thousand to 50 thousand yuan, and person(s) in charge and other directly responsible personnel be applied with disciplinary punishment; and in case crimes are committed, criminal liabilities shall be investigated and handled according to the law.

Article 44

In cases in which medical institutions undertake clinical trials or clinical verifications of medical devices and provide false reports, which violates provisions of these Regulations, the drug regulatory authority of governments at provincial level and above shall issue an order for correction and launch a warning, and may impose a fine of RM B 10 thousand to 30 thousand yuan;in serious cases, the qualification for clinical trial or clinical verification of medical devices shall be terminated, person(s) in charge and other directly responsible personnel shall receive disciplinary punishment; an d in case crimes are committed, criminal liability shall be investigated and handled according to the law.

Article 45

For cases in which testing institutions and their personnel are found to be conducting or involved in research and development, manufacturing, distribution and technical consultation of medical devices which are related to the testing, or establishing false testing reports, which violates provisions of these Regulations, the drug regulatory authority of governments at provincial level and above shall issue an order for correction and launch a warning, and may impose a fine of RMB 10 thousand to 30 thousand yuan; in serious cases, the qualification for testing shall be terminated by the drug regulatory authority under the State Council, person(s) in charge and other directly responsible personnel shall be receive disciplinary punishment; and in case crimes are committed, criminal liability shall be investigated and handled according to law.

Article 46

In cases where personnel engaged in supervision and administration of medical devices abuse their power, pursue personal benefits by deceiving, or neglecting their duties, in violation of provisions of these Regulations, to the extent to which crimes are committed, criminal liabilities shall be investigated and handled according to the law. For those not committing crimes, disciplinary punishment shall be applied according to the relevant regulations.

VI. SUPPLEMENTARY PROVISIONS

Article 47

Provisions governing non-profitable contraceptive devices shall be formulated separately by the drug regulatory authority in conjunction with other relevant authorities under the State Council.

Article 48

These Regulations shall come into force from April 1, 2000.

5

Health Authorities Acts and Rules

REGIONAL HEALTH AUTHORITIES ACT, NEW BRUWISWICK, CANADA

Her Majesty, by and with the advice and consent of the Legislative Assembly of New Brunswick, enacts as follows:

PART I: INTERPRETATION

Definitions

1. In this Act

"addiction services" means prevention, treatment or rehabilitation services provided to a patient affected by a drug, alcohol or gambling dependency; (« services de toxicomanie »)

"board" means a board of directors of a regional health authority; (« conseil »)

"community health centre" means a place in which community health services are delivered or provided; (« centre de santé communautaire »)

"community health services" means medical services and nursing or nurse practitioner services, and may include such other health services as are prescribed by regulation; (« services de santé communautaires »)

"extra-mural services" means acute, long term,

rehabilitative or palliative care provided to a patient at the patient's place of residence, place of work or other place in a community; (« services extra-muraux »)

"facility" means a building or premises in or from which health services are provided; (« établissement »)

"health region" means a health region established under section 15; (« région de la santé »)

"health services" means hospital services, addiction services, mental health services, public health services, extra-mural services and community health services; (« services de santé »)

"Minister" means the Minister of Health and includes any person designated by the Minister to act on behalf of the Minister; (« Ministre »)

"patient" means a person who receives health services from a regional health authority; (« malade »)

"provincial health plan" means the provincial health plan established, or amended, by the Minister under section 6; (« plan provincial de la santé »)

"public health services" means services provided to patients or members of the public through programs relating to sexuality, healthy lifestyles and immunization, and includes such other services as may be prescribed by regulation;

"regional health authority" means a regional health authority established under section 16; (« régie régionale de la santé »)

"regional health and business plan" means a plan approved or amended under section 32. (« plan régional de la sante et d'affaires »)

2002, c.40, s.1; 2004, c.16, s.3; 2006, c.16, s.159.

Purpose

2. The purpose of this Act is to establish regional health authorities with responsibility for providing for the delivery of and administering health services in specified geographic areas and, where authorized, in other areas of the Province.

Conflict

3 Where there is a conflict between this Act or the regulations and the Hospital Act or regulations under that Act, the provisions of this Act and the regulations prevail.

PART II: POWERS AND DUTIES OF THE MINISTER

Administration of Act

4(1) The Minister is responsible for the administration of this Act.

Designation by Minister

4(2) The Minister may designate one or more persons to act on the Minister's behalf.

Delegation by Minister

5. The Minister may delegate, in writing, any authority, power, duty or function conferred or imposed on the Minister under this Act to a regional health authority.

Provincial Health Plan

6(1) The Minister shall establish, and may amend, a provincial health plan, which shall include

(a) the principles upon which the provision of health services in the province are to be based,

(b) the provincial objectives and priorities for the provision of health services in the Province or areas of the Province,

(c) the health services to be provided or made available

by a regional health authority within its region and, where applicable, outside of its region,

(d) the health services to be acquired by the Minister from outside of the Province,

(e) the provincial programs for the provision of health services in the province,

(f) the nature and scope of any basic or applied research initiatives that are to be conducted in relation to health care and health services,

(g) the programs for training of persons in the medical and other health professions, including practice settings for the training of health professionals,

(h) the policy framework, parameters and standards for the consolidation of clinical and non-clinical services provided by regional health authorities,

(i) a comprehensive financial plan that includes a statement of how material and human resources, including but not limited to, financial resources, are to be allocated to meet the provincial health plan, and

(j) any other matter prescribed by regulation.

6(2) When establishing or amending the provincial health plan, the Minister shall have regard to the requirements of the Hospital Services Act.

6(3) The Minister shall consult with every regional health authority when preparing the provincial health plan, and when amending the provincial health plan.

Accountability Framework

7(1) The Minister shall establish an accountability framework that describes the roles of the Minister and other government ministers and the regional health authorities and that specifies the responsibilities each has towards the other within the provincial health system.

7(2) The Minister shall consult with every regional health authority when establishing an accountability framework.

Minister May Give Directions

8(1) The Minister may give directions to a regional health authority for the purpose of

(a) implementing the provincial health plan,

(b) providing priorities and guidelines for a regional health authority to follow in carrying out and exercising its responsibilities, duties and powers, and

(c) coordinating the work of the regional health authorities with each other and with the programs, policies and work of the government and other persons in the provision of health services.

8(2) The Minister may establish parameters and give directions to a regional health authority in relation to the planning, organization, management and delivery of health services by the regional health authority.

Minister May Establish Performance Targets

9. The Minister may establish performance targets for a regional health authority with respect to

(a) its development as an organization,

(b) its financial management,

(c) ensuring access to the health services provided by the regional health authority,

(d) achieving satisfactory patient outcomes,

(e) the level of patient satisfaction with the services provided by the regional health authority, and

(f) any other matter prescribed by regulation.

Provincial Standards for Health Services

10. The Minister may establish provincial standards for the provision of health services in the province and regions of the province and with respect to the quality of health services provided.

Health Services Provided by the Minister

11. Notwithstanding any provision of this or any other Act, where the Minister considers it in the public interest to do so, the Minister may

(a) provide or arrange for the provision of health services in an area of the province, or outside the province, whether or not the services are being provided by a regional health authority, and

(b) may do any other thing that the Minister considers necessary to ensure the provision of health services in the province.

Approval by Minister

12(1) The Minister may make an approval given by the Minister under this Act or the regulations subject to such terms and conditions as the Minister considers appropriate.

12(2) The Minister may suspend or revoke an approval given under this Act or the regulations.

Agreements by Minister

13. The Minister may enter into, and amend, agreements for the purposes of this Act with

(a) the government of Canada or of another province, territory or jurisdiction,

(b) a department, agency or body under the jurisdiction of the government of Canada or of another province, territory or jurisdiction,

(c) a band council as defined in the Indian Act (Canada),

(d) a regional health authority,

(e) a municipality or rural community, or

(f) or any other person or group of persons.

2005, c.7, s.74.

Review by Minister

14(1) The Minister shall ensure that a comprehensive review is commenced within five years after the commencement of this Act for the purpose of examining and reporting on the effectiveness of moving to a regional health authority system.

14(2) The Minister shall ensure that a review under subsection (1) is concluded no later than eighteen months after it commences.

14(3) The Minister shall lay the report prepared as a result of the review before the Legislative Assembly within thirty days after receiving the report, or if the Legislative Assembly is not sitting, when it next sits.

PART III: REGIONAL HEALTH AUTHORITIES

DIVISION A: ESTABLISHMENT OF HEALTH REGIONS AND REGIONAL HEALTH AUTHORITIES

Establishment of Health Regions

15(1) The regions described and named in Schedule A are established as health regions for the purposes of this Act.

15(2) The Lieutenant-Governor in Council may, by regulation, vary the boundaries of a health region.

Establishment of Regional Health Authorities

16. There are established the following regional health authorities for the health regions listed below:

(a) two regional health authorities for Health Region 1, one to be known as Regional Health Authority 1(Beauséjour)/ Régie régionale de la santé 1 (Beauséjour) and the other as Regional Health Authority 1(South-East)/Régie régionale de la santé 1 (sud-est);

(b) one regional health authority for Health Region 2, to be known as Regional Health Authority 2/Régie régionale de la santé 2;

(c) one regional health authority for Health Region 3, to be known as Regional Health Authority 3/Régie régionale de la santé 3;

(d) one regional health authority for Health Region 4, to be known as Regional Health Authority 4/Régie régionale de la santé 4;

(e) one regional health authority for Health Region 5, to be known as Regional Health Authority 5/Régie régionale de la santé 5;

(f) one regional health authority for Health Region 6, to be known as Regional Health Authority 6/Régie régionale de la santé 6;

(g) one regional health authority for Health Region 7, to be known as Regional Health Authority 7/Régie régionale de la santé 7.

Legal Status of Regional Health Authority

17. A regional health authority is a body corporate and,

subject to this Act and the regulations, has all the rights, powers and privileges of a natural person of full capacity for the purposes of carrying out and exercising its responsibilities, duties and powers under this Act.

Non-profit Body Corporate

18. A regional health authority is established to operate exclusively as a body corporate without share capital, and no part of the income or property of a regional health authority shall be paid to, or otherwise be made available for, the personal benefit of any director of the authority.

DIVISION B: STRUCTURE AND ADMINISTRATION

Board of Regional Health Authority

19(1) The business and affairs of a regional health authority shall be controlled and managed by a board of directors, appointed or elected in accordance with this Act and the regulations.

Directions of Minister to Board

19(2) Notwithstanding subsection (1), where the Minister is of the opinion that a decision of a board is inconsistent with its regional health and business plan, the Minister may override the decision of the board and substitute his or her decision for that of the board to ensure compliance with the plan, and the decision of the Minister shall be deemed to be the decision of the board.

19(3) Notwithstanding subsection (1), where the Minister is of the opinion that a board of a regional health authority has failed or is failing to ensure compliance with the regional health and business plan for the regional health authority, the Minister may give directions in respect of the matter, and the directions of the Minister shall be deemed to be the directions of the board.

19(4) Where the Minister makes a decision under subsection (2) or gives a direction under subsection (3), the chief executive officer shall ensure that the decisions and directions of the Minister are carried out.

Composition of Board

19(5) A board of a regional health authority shall consist of fifteen voting members and three non-voting members as follows:

(a) seven voting members who shall be appointed by the Minister;
(b) eight voting members who shall be elected;
(c) the chief executive officer, who shall be a non-voting member;
(d) the chairperson of the professional advisory committee, who shall be a non-voting member; and
(e) the chairperson of the medical advisory committee, who shall be a non-voting member.

Quorum

19(6) A majority of the voting members of the board constitutes a quorum.

Vacancy

19(7) A vacancy on the board does not impair the capacity of the board to act.

19(8) Where a vacancy occurs on the board, the Minister may appoint a person to fill the vacancy for the balance of the term of the member replaced.

Disqualification of board member

19(9) Where a board member is disqualified from holding office as a member of the board, the remaining members of the board shall declare the office to be vacant and shall immediately notify the Minister of that fact.

Chairperson

19(11) The chairperson of the board shall be selected in accordance with the by-laws.

Remuneration and Expenses of Directors

19(12) A regional health authority shall pay its directors such remuneration and expenses as the Lieutenant-Governor in Council determines.

First Directors

20(1) Notwithstanding subsection 19(1), the first board of directors of a regional health authority shall consist of

(a) fifteen voting members appointed by the Minister, and

(b) the three non-voting members referred to in paragraphs 19(5)(c) to (e).

20(2) The Minister may

(a) notwithstanding subsection 19(11), appoint one of the first directors as the first chairperson of the board of the regional health authority, and

(b) make subsequent appointments to fill vacancies on the board until directors are appointed or elected under subsection 19(1), and a person appointed under this paragraph is deemed to be a first director.

20(3) The terms of office of a first director and first chairperson of a regional health authority continue until their successors are appointed or elected under subsection 19(1).

By-laws and Policies

21(1) A board shall make by-laws and policies not inconsistent with this Act regarding its internal organization and proceedings and for the general conduct and management of the affairs of the regional health authority.

21(2) The by-laws made by a board, and all amendments to them, shall be submitted to the Minister for approval in accordance with the procedures established by the Minister.

21(3) A by-law of a board has no force and effect until approved by the Minister.

21(4) A regional health authority shall ensure that its by-laws are available for inspection by members of the public during normal office hours.

Meetings of the Board

22(1) A member of the board of directors of a regional health authority shall not vote by proxy at a meeting of the board of directors.

22(2) A member of the board of directors of a regional health authority may participate in a meeting of the board of directors or of a committee of the board of directors by means of telephone or other communication facilities that permit all persons participating in the meeting to hear each other if

(a) the by-laws of the regional health authority so provide, or

(b) subject to the by-laws, all members of the board of directors consent.

22(3) A member of a board of directors participating in a meeting in accordance with subsection (2) shall be deemed to be present at the meeting.

23(1) Subject to subsection (2), a board shall hold its meetings open to the public.

23(2) A board may hold a meeting, or a portion of a meeting, in private if, in the board's opinion, the meeting or portion of the meeting would

(a) reveal information specific to an identifiable individual,

(b) reveal information relating to risk management issues or patient care issues,

(c) prejudice any security measures undertaken by the regional health authority, or

(d) compromise the regional health authority's effectiveness in carrying out its duties and responsibilities.

Minutes

24(1) A board shall ensure that the minutes of each meeting are recorded.

24(2) Where a board holds a meeting, or a portion of a meeting, in private, it shall ensure that the minutes of the meeting indicate the nature of the subject matter to be discussed in private and why the board, in its opinion, considers it necessary to hold the meeting, or portion of the meeting, in private.

24(3) A board shall forward a copy of the adopted minutes of a meeting to the Minister within seven days after the meeting at which the minutes were adopted, and shall provide the Minister with the minutes of any meeting, or portion of the meeting, that was held in private.

24(4) A board shall ensure that the adopted minutes, other than the minutes arising from a meeting or portion of the meeting that was held in private, are made available to the public during normal business hours.

Conflict of Interest

25(1) A member of a board shall not vote on or speak to a matter before the board if

(a) the member has an interest in the matter, distinct from an interest arising from his or her functions as a member,

(b) the member has a direct or indirect pecuniary interest in the matter,

(c) a parent, spouse, brother, sister or child of the member has an interest in the matter, or

(d) the member is an officer, employee or agent of a corporation or an unincorporated association, or other association of persons that has an interest in the matter.

25(2) Where a member is in conflict, the member shall disclose to the board the nature and extent of the interest either in writing or by requesting to have it entered in the minutes of the meeting of the board.

25(3) A member shall disclose a conflict of interest

(a) at the meeting where the matter giving rise to the conflict of interest is considered, or

(b) if the member is not in a conflict of interest at the time described in paragraph (a), at the first meeting that is held after the conflict arises.

Chief Executive Officer

26(1) Notwithstanding subsection 6(2) of the Financial Administration Act, the Deputy Minister of the Department of Health shall, with respect to a chief executive officer of a regional health authority, be deemed to be the delegate of the Board of Management for the purpose of appointing and terminating the appointment of, and for setting the terms and conditions of employment a chief executive officer within the parameters set by the Board of Management.

26(2) The chief executive officer of a regional health

authority shall report to the Deputy Minister of the Department of Health.

26(3) Notwithstanding that an appointment is made under subsection (1), and notwithstanding subsection (2), the position of chief executive officer of a regional health authority shall be deemed in Part III of the public service of the Province as specified in the First Schedule of the Public Service Labour Relations Act for the purpose of all other matters that relate to the employment relationship.

26(4) The chief executive officer is responsible for the general management and conduct of the affairs of the regional health authority within the by-laws, policies and directions of the board.

2006, c.16, s.159.

Professional Advisory Committee

27(1) A board shall, in accordance with the by-laws, establish a professional advisory committee to advise the board respect to

(a) clinical care and health issues,
(b) criteria for admission and discharge of patients,
(c) quality assurance and risk management with respect to the health services delivered by the regional health authority, and
(d) any other issues the board may refer to the committee.

27(2) A professional advisory committee shall consist of not more than fifteen members appointed by the board, at least five of whom shall be members of different health professions that are self-regulated under a private Act.

Medical Advisory Committee

28(1) A board shall, in accordance with the by-laws, establish a medical advisory committee.

(a) to advise the board with respect to appointments to the medical staff and on privileges of members of the medical staff, and

(b) to investigate, at the request of the board, questions requiring medical judgment and to report to the board.

28(2) Before making appointments to the medical staff of a regional health authority or granting privileges, a board of directors shall request advice from the medical advisory committee as to the appointments to be made and the privileges to be granted.

28(3) A medical advisory committee shall make adequate provision for the supervision of all medical services and dental services provided by a regional health authority.

DIVISION C: POWERS, DUTIES AND RESPONSIBILITIES OF REGIONAL HEALTH AUTHORITIES

Responsibilities of Regional Health Authority

29(1) A regional health authority shall provide for the delivery of and administer health services in the region for which it is established.

29(2) Notwithstanding subsection (1), a regional health authority may, where authorized under its regional health and business plan, deliver health services in another region.

Determination of Health Needs

30. A regional health authority shall

(a) determine the health needs of the population that it serves,

(b) determine the priorities in the provision of health services for the population it serves, and

(c) allocate resources according to the regional health and business plan.

Provision of Health Services

31. A regional health authority may provide health services only where

(a) there is a need for health services,

(b) the services are included in a plan approved by the Minister,

(c) the services are consistent with the provincial health plan, and

(d) sufficient resources are available.

Regional Health and Business Plan

32(1) A regional health authority shall, within the time and form specified by the Minister, prepare and submit to the Minister a proposed regional health and business plan that, having regard to the provincial health plan, includes

(a) the principles upon which the provision of health services by the regional health authority are to be based,

(b) the objectives and priorities of the regional health authority for the provision of health services to meet the health needs in the health region and, where applicable, to meet the health needs of persons in other parts of the Province,

(c) the health services to be delivered and administered by the regional health authority and where the services are to be provided,

(d) the nature and scope of any basic or applied research initiatives in relation to health care and health services,

(e) the programs for training of persons in the medical and other health professions, including practice settings for the training of health professionals.

THE CENTRAL MENTAL HEALTH AUTHORITY RULES 1990, INDIA

G.S.R. 1004 (E) DATED 20TH DECEMBER 1990.1 - In exercise of the powers conferred by sub-section (1) of Sec. 94 of the Mental Health Act, 1987, (14 of 1987), read with Sec. 22 of the General Clauses Act, 1897 (10 of 1897), the Central Government hereby makes the following rules, namely:

I. PRELIMINARY

1. Short Title and Commencement

1. These rules may be called the Central Mental Health Authority Rules, 1990.
2. They shall come into force on the date of commencement of the Act.

2. Definitions

In these rules unless the context otherwise requires -

(a) "Act" means the Mental Health Act, 1987 (14 of 1987);

(b) "Authority" means the Central Mental Health Authority established under Sec. 3 of the Act;

(c) "Chairman" means the Chairman nominated under rule 5;

(d) "Member" means member of the Authority appointed under rule 3.

(e) "Membership" means the membership of the Authority established under rule 3.

(f) "Non-Official Member" means a member appointed under sub-rule (2) of rule3;

(g) "Official Member" means a member appointed under sub-rule (1) of rule3;

(h) "Secretary" means the Secretary to the Authority appointed under rule 13;

(i) Words and expressions used herein and not defined but defined in the Act shall respectively have the meaning assigned to them in the Act.

II. CENTRAL MENTAL HEALTH AUTHORITY

3. Constitution of the Authority

The Authority shall consist of the following members, namely;

1. Official Member -
   - (a) Secretary or Additional Secretary, Ministry of Health and Family Welfare, Government of India.
   - (b) Joint Secretary, Ministry of Health and Family Welfare dealing with Mental Health.
   - (c) Additional Director-General of Health Services dealing with Mental Health.
   - (d) Director, Central Institute of Psychiatry,Ranchi.
   - (e) Director, National Institute of Mental Health and Neuro Sciences,Bangalore.
   - (f) Medical Superintendent, Hospital for Mental diseases, Shahdara, Delhi.
2. Non-Official Members- Three members including one social Worker, one clinical psychologist and one Medical psychiatric who, in the opinion of the central Government, have speical interest in the field of Mental Health.

Comment

This rule provides that the Authority under this rule shall consist of certain official and non-official members mentioned therein.

4. Disqulification

A persons shall be disqualification for being appointed as a members or shall be removed from membership by the Central Government if he,-

(a) has been convicted and sentenced to imprisonment for an offence which in the opinion of the Central Government involves moral turpitude ; or

(b) is an undischarged insolvent;or

(c) is of unsound mind and stands so declared by a competent court, or

(d) has been removed or dismissed from the Government or a body corporate owned or controlled by the Government.

5. Chairman

1. The Central Government may nominate any official member to act as the Chairman of the Authority.
2. The Chairman shall cease to hold office when he ceases to be a member of the Authority.

6. Term Office of Members

1. Every official member shall hold office as such member so long as he holds the office by virtue of which he was appointed.
2. Every non-official member shall hold office for a period of three years from the date of his appointment and shall be eligible for re-appointment.

3. A non-official member may at any time resign from membership of the Authority by forwarding his letter of resignation to the Chairman and such resignation shall take effect only from the date on which it is accepted.
4. Where a vacancy occurs by resignation of a non-official member under sub-rule (3) or otherwise, the Central Government shall fill the vacancy by appointing from amongst category of persons referred to in sub-clause (2) of rule 3 and the person so appointed, shall hold office for the remainder of the term of office of the member in whose place he was so appointed.
5. Where the term of office of any non-official member is about to expire the Central Government may appointment a successor at any time within three months before the expiry of the term of such member but the successor shall not assume office until the term of the member expires.

III. PROCEEDINGS OF THE AUTHORITY

7. Meetings of the Authority

1. The authority shall ordinarily meet once in every six months at such time and place as may be fixed by the Chairman. Provided that the Chairman -
   (i) May call a special meeting at any time to deal with any urgent matter requiring the attention of the Authority.
   (ii) Shall call a special meeting if he receives a requisition in writing signed by not less than four members and stating the purpose for which they desire the meeting to be called.
2. The first meeting of the Authority to be held in any

calendar year shall be the annual meeting for that year.

8. Subjects for Special Meeting

Where a meeting referred to in the proviso to sub-rule (1) of rule 7 has been convened, only the subjects for the consideration of which the meeting was convened, shall be discussed.

9. Subjects for the Annual Meeting

At the Annual Meeting of the Authority, the following subjects shall be considered and disposed of namely;-

1. Review of the progress of implementation of the various provisions of Mental Health Act during the preceding one year.
2. Other business on the agenda; and
3. Any other business brought forward with the consent of the Chairman or where he is absent, with the consent of officer presiding at the meeting.

10. Procedure for Holding Meetings

1. Every notice calling for a meeting of the authority shall - specify the place, date and hour of the meeting:
   (a) Be served upon every member of the Authority not less than twenty-one clear days in the case of annual meeting and fiteen clear days in the case of other meetings before the day appointed for the meeting.
2. The Secretary shall prepare and circulate to the members alongwith the notice of the meeting an agenda for such meeting showing the business to be transacted.
3. A member who wishes to move a resolution on any matter included in the agenda shall give notice

thereof to the Secretary not less than seven days before the date fixed for the meeting.

4. A member who wishes to move any motion not included in the agenda shall give notice to the Secretary not less than fourteen days before the date fixed for the meeting.

Comment

This rule lays down the procedure for holding the meeting.

11. Proceedings of the Authority

1. The Chairman or in his absence any member authorised by him shall preside at the meetings of the Authority.
2. The quorum for the meeting of the Authority shall be four members.
3. If within half an hour from time appointed for holding a meeting of th Authority quorum is not present, the meeting shall be adjourned to the same day in the following week at the same time and place and the presiding officer of such meeting shall inform the members present and send notice to other members.
4. If at the adjourned meeting also, quorum is not present within half an hour from the time appointed for holding the meeting, the members present shall constitute the quorum.
5. In the adjourned meeting if the Chairman is not present and no member has been authorised to preside at such meeting, the members present shall elect a member to preside at the meeting.
6. Each member including the Chairman shall have one vote. In the case of an equality of votes, the Chairman or any member presiding over such meeting shall in addition, have a casting vote.

7. All decisions of the meeting of the Authority shall be taken by a majority of the members present and voting.

12. Approval by Circulation

Any business which may be necessary for the Authority to transact except as such may be placed before the annual meeting, may be circulated and approved by a majority of members, shall be valid and binding as if such resolution had been passed at the meeting of the Authority.

13. Secretary of the Authority

1. The Chairman shall cause to be appointed a Secretary to the Authority from amongst persons possessing post-graduate degree in psychiatry and having three years' experience in the field of psychiatry.
2. The Secretary shall be a full-time or part-time servant of the Authority and shall function as the Administrative Officer of the Authority.
3. The Secretary shall be responsible for the control and management of office accounts and correspondence.
4. The Secretary shall cause to be appointed such members of the ministerial and non-ministerial staff which are essential for the efficient functioning of the Authority.
5. The Secretary shall exercise such other powers and discharge such other functions as may be authorised in writing by the Chairman for the efficient functioning of the Authority.

14. Forwarding of Copies of the Proceedings of the Authority to to the Central Government

The Secretary shall forward copies of the proceedings of the Authority to the Central Government periodically.

6

Hospital and Health Insurance Acts

HOSPITAL INSURANCE ACT, VICTORIA, BRITISH COLUMBIA, CANADA

[RSBC 1996] Chapter 2004

Definitions

1. In this Act:

"beneficiary" means a beneficiary as defined in section 1 of the *Medicare Protection Act;*

"benefits" means the general hospital services authorized under this Act;

"hospital" means, except in sections 24 and 29 (2) (a),

(a) a hospital as defined by section 1 of the *Hospital Act* that has been designated under this Act by the Lieutenant Governor in Council as a hospital required to provide the general hospital services provided under this Act,

(b) a private hospital as defined by section 5 of the *Hospital Act* with which the government has entered into an agreement requiring the hospital to provide the general hospital services provided under this Act,

(c) a hospital owned and operated by Canada that has been designated under this Act a "federal hospital",

(d) an agency or establishment that

(i) provides a service to hospitals or a health service and

(ii) has been designated as a hospital facility by the Lieutenant Governor in Council, or

(e) an establishment in which out patient services are available that has been designated a diagnostic and treatment centre by the Lieutenant Governor in Council for providing out patient benefits to beneficiaries in accordance with this Act and the regulations;

"Nisga'a Nation" has the same meaning as in the Nisga'a Final Agreement;

"PHSA" means the Provincial Health Services Authority, a society incorporated under the *Society Act;*

"regional health board" means a board as defined in section 1 of the *Health Authorities Act;*

"resident" means a resident as defined in section 1 of the *Medicare Protection Act.*

Repealed

2 [Repealed 2002-16-2.]

Beneficiaries

3 (1) Subject to this Act and the regulations, every beneficiary is entitled to receive the general hospital services provided under this Act.

(2) [Repealed 2002-16-3.]

Benefits for Beneficiaries Only

4 No person other than a beneficiary is entitled to the benefits provided by this Act.

Benefits

5 (1) Except as provided in subsection (2), the general hospital services provided under this Act are the following:

(a) for beneficiaries requiring treatment for acute illness or injury, the public ward accommodation, necessary operating and case room facilities, diagnostic or therapeutic X-ray and laboratory procedures, anesthetics, prescriptions, drugs, dressings, cast materials and other services prescribed by regulation;

(b) for beneficiaries requiring active treatment for chronic illness or disability, the public ward accommodation, physiotherapy and occupational therapy, minor operating room and diagnostic X-ray and laboratory services, prescriptions, drugs, dressings, cast materials and other services prescribed by regulation;

(c) for beneficiaries requiring treatment or diagnostic services as out patients, the out patient treatment or diagnostic services prescribed by regulation.

(2) General hospital services under this Act do not include the following:

(a) transportation to or from hospital;

(b) services or treatment that the minister, or a person designated by the minister, determines, on a review of the medical evidence, the beneficiary does not require;

(c) services or treatment for an illness or condition excluded by regulation of the Lieutenant Governor in Council.

(3) For the purposes of subsection (1) (c), the regulations may authorize the minister to define categories of out patient care and specify the treatment or diagnostic services to be provided for those categories.

(4) No person is entitled to receive any of the benefits under this Act unless

(a) it has been certified in the manner provided in the regulations that the person requires the services, and

(b) it is proved to the satisfaction of the minister that the person is a beneficiary.

(5) [Repealed 2002-16-5.]

(6) If a person does not obtain certification as provided in subsection (4), the person has no claim against the government for general hospital services provided to the person.

(7) Subject to the approval of the Lieutenant Governor in Council, the right of a beneficiary to receive the benefits under this Act may be made subject to the payment by or on behalf of the beneficiary of a portion of the cost of providing any treatment or services rendered to the beneficiary by a hospital, and the government must pay, on behalf of any person who is certified by the minister charged by order of the Lieutenant Governor in Council with the administration of the *Employment and Assistance Act* to be a person entitled to health services, a charge levied under this subsection against that person.

Payment for Organ Donor not a Beneficiary

6 Despite this Act, if a beneficiary requires an organ transplant from a donor who is not a beneficiary, the cost of diagnosis, services and treatment rendered to the donor by

the hospital must be paid to the hospital in a manner and amount the minister directs.

Necessary Information to be Supplied on Request

7 (1) The minister or an officer of the Ministry of Health or of a hospital may require a person to provide, by means of an affidavit or otherwise, information regarding the person or the members of the person's family thought necessary by the minister or an officer for the proper administration of this Act.

(2) A person who does any of the following commits an offence:

(a) makes a false statement of fact in an affidavit or statement required under this Act;

(b) fails or refuses to make an affidavit or statement at once on being required to do so;

(c) withholds or misrepresents information regarding a matter connected with this Act.

(3) A person who commits an offence under subsection (2) is liable on conviction to a penalty of not less than $100 or to imprisonment for not less than 10 days, or both.

Hospitals to Provide Services for Beneficiaries

8 Every hospital must provide for beneficiaries those public ward facilities, including necessary operating and case room facilities, X-ray and laboratory diagnostic and therapeutic procedures, anesthetics, and other services, dressings and drugs the Lieutenant Governor in Council requires or provides for under regulations.

Payment to a regional health board, the Nisga'a Nation or the PHSA

9 (1) There must be paid annually to

(a) each regional health board,

(b) the Nisga'a Nation, and

(c) the PHSA

For the hospitals it funds an amount determined by the minister to cover all or part of the cost to the regional health board, the Nisga'a Nation or the PHSA for the provision to beneficiaries of those general hospital services authorized by this Act that the hospitals are required by the minister to provide for beneficiaries admitted for treatment, excluding those amounts payable for those hospitals under section 5 (7) and section 14.

(2) The fiscal year of a hospital begins April 1.

Nonbeneficiaries

10 (1) The government is not liable for payment of the cost of providing any hospital service or treatment rendered to a person who is not a beneficiary.

(2) [Repealed 2003-33-6.]

(3) Despite a contract or any other Act, payment for hospital services or treatment rendered to a person who is not a beneficiary must be made to the hospital by the person or on the person's behalf.

(4) For the purposes of subsection (3),

(a) the hospital must compute the amount owing by or on behalf of that person in a manner approved by the minister, and

(b) each computation must be based on the rate or charge approved by the minister.

(5) If a patient is not a beneficiary, the hospital has a cause of action against the patient or the person legally

liable to pay for the hospital services or treatment rendered to the patient for the amount owing in respect of them as determined under this section.

(6) For the purposes of subsection (5), if the patient claims to be entitled to benefits under this Act, the burden of proving that he or she is a beneficiary is on that person.

(7) If a person receives hospital services or treatment other than services or treatment authorized under this Act, payment of a sum computed by the hospital must be made to the hospital by or on behalf of that person for the cost of the other special services or treatment, in addition to the payment of other sums to which the hospital is entitled for any general hospital care which the hospital has rendered to that person.

Persons Who May be Excluded from Benefits

11. The Lieutenant Governor in Council may by regulation exclude, in whole or in part, from the benefits provided under this Act

(a) a person who is entitled to receive hospital care or treatment under an Act of Canada or of British Columbia specified in an agreement entered into between British Columbia and Canada, or

(b) a person who is entitled to receive hospital care or treatment from a government other than the government of British Columbia or of Canada.

A Regional Health Board, the Nisga'a Nation or the PHSA Must Not Seek Additional Payment

12. If a regional health board, the Nisga'a Nation or the PHSA has been paid by the government for general hospital services provided under this Act, the payment, subject to section 5 (7) or 14, is deemed to be payment in full for the services, and the regional health board, the Nisga'a Nation,

the PHSA or a hospital must not seek to recover additional payment from any other person for the services.

Offence to Bill Beneficiary for Insured Services

13. (1) A person wilfully rendering an account or causing an account to be rendered to a beneficiary for hospital services that are provided, and to which the beneficiary is entitled under this Act, commits an offence.

(2) A person who commits an offence under subsection (1) is liable on conviction to a fine of not more than $500.

Other than Public Ward Accommodation

14. (1) If a person entitled to the benefits provided by this Act requests and receives care in addition to public ward care, or if additional care is provided for a patient on the order of his or her physician,

(a) the hospital must be paid on the basis of public ward care as provided in this Act, and

(b) the hospital may collect from the patient and retain the difference in rates between the public ward care and the actual care provided.

(2) A proportion of all sums collected and retained by the hospitals under subsection (1) must be applied toward the cost of providing care in addition to public ward care.

(3) The proportion of the sums referred to in subsection (2) to be applied under that subsection must be in accordance with the directions issued by the minister.

Repealed

15 [Repealed RS1996 (Supp)-204-6.]

Accounting

16 The minister must keep accounts of the money received and expended under this Act.

Agreement with Other Governments

17 The minister may enter into an agreement with any other province

(a) to bring about a high degree of liaison and cooperation between the provinces concerning hospital insurance matters, and

(b) to make arrangements under which a beneficiary may move his or her home from one province to the other without ceasing to be entitled to benefits.

Other Agreements

18 The minister may enter into agreements with other agencies, associations, societies or companies for taking over commitments made by agencies providing for hospital care of certain individuals or groups resident in British Columbia.

Workers' Compensation Board

19 The Lieutenant Governor in Council may make regulations

(a) for coordinating the benefits available under the *Workers Compensation Act* with the general hospital services provided under this Act,

(b) for preventing duplication and difficulties in administration, and

(c) authorizing both the minister and the Workers' Compensation Board to enter into an agreement regulating their respective responsibilities and financial obligations.

Acquisition of Hospitals and Health Facilities

20 With the approval of the Lieutenant Governor in Council, the minister may

(a) acquire, including acquisition by expropriation, hospitals and health facilities, and land, buildings and equipment to be used for hospital or health facility purposes, and lease or transfer them to nonprofit agencies or corporations to be used as or for hospitals or health facilities, and

(b) enter into agreements for the purposes of paragraph (a).

Special Services

21 (1) The Lieutenant Governor in Council may provide for special or emergency aid in making available hospital services for particular parts or areas of British Columbia.

(2) [Repealed RS1996 (Supp)-204-8.]

Dispute as to whether services required

22 (1) If a dispute arises between a beneficiary and the minister as to whether the beneficiary requires hospital services, the beneficiary, if required by the minister, must submit himself or herself for examination by a medical practitioner appointed by the minister.

(2) If the beneficiary does not submit himself or herself for examination when required by the minister or if the beneficiary in any way obstructs an examination by the medical practitioner,

(a) his or her rights under this Act are suspended until the examination has taken place, and

(b) the beneficiary is personally liable for any hospital service received by him or her during the suspension.

Physician's Report

23 (1) The minister must secure reports the minister thinks necessary from the attending physician in a specific

case and may make payment to physicians for the reports.

(2) A physician commits an offence if he or she, having received notice by registered mail from the minister of information required by the physician, fails to comply with the notice.

(3) A physician who fails to make a report required by this Act or the regulations, unless excused by the minister, commits an offence.

(4) A person who commits an offence under subsection (2) or (3) is liable on conviction to a fine of not more than $50.

Hospital Services Outside British Columbia

24 Subject to this Act and the regulations, the minister must pay for hospital services rendered outside British Columbia to beneficiaries by

(a) hospitals, and

(b) other institutions

approved by the minister.

Third Party Liability

25 (1) If, as a result of the wrongful act or omission of another, a beneficiary suffers personal injuries for which the beneficiary receives hospital services paid for by the government, the beneficiary has the same right to recover the sum paid for the services against the person guilty of the wrongful act or omission as the beneficiary would have had, had the beneficiary been required to pay for the services personally.

(2) On the beneficiary recovering the sum or part of it under subsection (1), the beneficiary must pay it at once to the minister.

(3) The minister may order that a commission be paid for money recovered under subsection (1) and the amount of the commission and the conditions under which it may be paid must be in accordance with the rules prescribed by the Lieutenant Governor in Council.

(4) The government is subrogated to the rights of the beneficiary to recover sums paid for hospital services by the government, and an action may be maintained by the government, either its name or the name of the beneficiary, for the recovery of the sum paid for hospital services as provided in subsection (1).

(5) It is not a defence to an action brought by the government under subsection (4) that a claim for damages has been adjudicated on unless the claim included a claim for the sum paid for hospital services, and it is not a defence to an action brought by a beneficiary for damages for personal injuries that an action taken by the government under subsection (4) has been adjudicated on.

(6) No release or settlement of a claim or judgment based on a cause of action for damages for personal injuries in a case where the injured person has received hospital services paid for by the government is binding on the government unless the minister or a person designated by the minister has approved the settlement in writing.

(7) The Lieutenant Governor in Council may, by regulation, limit or define the circumstances that give rise to a cause of action under this section.

(8) This section applies to claims for hospital services arising after a day to be set by the Lieutenant Governor in Council.

Service of Notices

26 (1) Notice required to be given under this Act or the regulations

(a) must be in writing, and

(b) may be served by mailing it by prepaid post to the person named in it at the person's last known address.

(2) A person served with notice under subsection (1) is deemed to have received it on the day on which it would reach the person in the ordinary course of mail.

Penalties

27 If this Act, or regulations, rules or orders made under it by the Lieutenant Governor in Council are contravened, and no other penalty is provided for, the person guilty of the contravention is liable on conviction to a penalty of not more than $100 for each offence.

Limitation Period for Laying Charges

28 An information for an offence against this Act must be laid within 6 years from the time when the matter of the information arose.

Power to Make Regulations

29 (1) The Lieutenant Governor in Council may make regulations referred to in section 41 of the *Interpretation Act*.

(2) Without limiting this section, the Lieutenant Governor in Council may make regulations for the following:

(a) the amount and method of payment to hospitals and other institutions referred to in section 24 for hospital services rendered outside British Columbia to beneficiaries under this Act and the number of days of care for which payment will be made to those hospitals and other institutions;

(b) the facilities and services that a regional health board, the Nisga'a Nation or the PHSA must provide for beneficiaries under this Act in order to qualify them for payment by the government, and the amount of the payment to regional health boards, the Nisga'a Nation or the PHSA;

(c) [Repealed 2002-16-8.]

(d) the manner and form in which reports must be made and accounts rendered to the minister, and all other matters and procedures concerned with payment of accounts or their compilation and presentation;

(e) inquiries to determine the correctness of accounts rendered by hospitals, regional health boards, the Nisga'a Nation or the PHSA;

(f) the treatment and services referred to in section 5;

(g) the kind of information to be obtained under this Act;

(h) the presentation by the board of management of a hospital of satisfactory medical certification to show clearly the need of any patient for hospital care and treatment;

(i) the length of stay in a hospital for which payment may be made by the government on behalf of a beneficiary;

(j) the acquisition or use of land as sites for hospitals, and the creation, establishment, construction, alteration, equipment, maintenance and repair of hospitals;

(k) the provision of any special or other type of service for any particular area that the Lieutenant Governor in Council may provide;

(l) the classification, grades and standards of hospitals;

(m) the inspection, control, government, management, conduct, operation and use of hospitals;

(n) the exclusion of persons, in whole or in part, from the benefits provided under this Act;

(o) the admission, treatment, conduct, discipline and discharge of patients;

(p) the records, books, accounting systems, audits, reports and returns to be made and kept by hospitals;

(q) morbidity reporting by hospitals;

(r) communicable diseases, tuberculosis and maternity patients;

(s) the equipment and use of laboratory, X-ray and operating and case rooms;

(t) the records, books, accounting systems, audits, reports and returns to be made and kept by the minister;

(u) [Repealed RS1996 (Supp)-204-11.]

(v) the kind of information that must be considered confidential and need not be divulged;

(w) financial aid to institutions approved under the *Hospital Act;*

(x) certification of requirements for admission to hospital;

(y) the information that associations, companies or other agencies engaged in providing hospital insurance must provide to the minister;

(z) definitions of expressions not defined elsewhere in this Act.

(3) Without limiting this section, the Lieutenant Governor in Council may make regulations for the following:

(a) provision for the payment by or on behalf of a

beneficiary of a portion of the cost of providing any treatment or services rendered to the beneficiary by a hospital and the manner in which the payment is to be calculated and made;

(b) the exemption of persons or classes of persons from making payments referred to in paragraph (a);

(c) payment of a commission for money recovered under section 25;

(d) securing information from persons living in British Columbia thought necessary by the minister for the administration of this Act, the prescribing of forms by the minister for this purpose, and prescribing rules for the use of the forms;

(e) the establishment of advisory committees and boards with objects and powers that appear advisable, and the appointment and remuneration of the members.

7

Health Care Laws

MASSACHUSETTS USA

Acts of 2006 of the Massachusetts Legislature: An Act Providing Access to Affordable, Quality, Accountable Health Care is a legislative provision from 2006 designed to extend health care coverage to all of the residents of Massachusetts, U.S.A.

Background

As of March, 2006 there were around 500,000 uninsured residents of Massachusetts. Those who are uninsured commonly utilize emergency rooms as a source of primary care because of their lack of insurance coverage. Massachusetts hospitals are required to provide care even if a patient cannot pay for it. As a result, hospitals have been left with unpaid bills and mounting expenses to care for the uninsured.

In Massachusetts, an approximately $600 million fund known as the Uncompensated Care Pool (or "free care pool") is used to partially reimburse hospitals and health centers for these expenses. The fund is raised through an annual assessment on insurance providers and hospitals, plus contributions of state and federal tax revenue. MIT professor Jonathan Gruber studied the state's population and health care needs and determined that there was enough money in the "free care pool" to pay for reform legislation without requiring additional funding or taxes.

In November 2004, political leaders began advocating for major reforms of the Massachusetts health care system to expand coverage. First, the Senate President Robert Travaglini called for a plan to reduce the number of uninsured by half. A few days later, the Governor, Mitt Romney, announced that he would propose a plan to cover virtually all of the uninsured.

At the same time, a broad coalition of health activists introduced a bill that expanded MassHealth (Medicaid) coverage, increased health coverage subsidy programmes and required employers to either provide coverage or pay an assessment to the state. The coalition stated they would gather signatures to place their proposal on the ballot in November 2006 if the legislature did not enact comprehensive health access reform. The Blue Cross Blue Shield Foundation also sponsored a study, "Roadmap to Coverage," that set out a number of methods to expand coverage to everyone in the Commonwealth.

The state also faced pressure from the federal government, which insisted that changes be made to the federal waiver that allows Massachusetts to operate an expanded Medicaid programme. Under the existing waiver, the state was receving $385 million in federal funds to assist health plans operated for the uninsured by two public hospital systems. The federal authorities directed the state to shift those funds to insurance coverage.

These forces converged in fall 2005 as the House and Senate passed health reform bills that drew on proposals of the Governor, the activist coalition, and legislative initiatives.

The legislature made a number of changes to Governor

Romney's original proposal, including expanding MassHealth (Medicaid) coverage to low-income children and restoring funding for public health programmes. The most controversial change was adding a provision charging firms with 11 or more workers that do not provide "fair and reasonable" health coverage to their workers. The charge, initially $295 annually per worker, is intended to equalize the free care pool charges imposed on employers who do and do not cover their workers. The legislature also rejected Governor Romney's proposal to permit high-deductible, low benefit health plans.

On April 12, 2006 Governor Mitt Romney signed the health legislation. He vetoed 8 sections of the health care legislation, including the employer assessment. Romney also vetoed provisions providing dental benefits to poor residents on the Medicaid programme, and providing health coverage to senior and disabled legal immigrants not eligible for federal Medicaid.

The legislature overrode all of the eight gubernatorial vetoes. On May 1, 2006, the Commonwealth submitted its implementation plan to the federal government.

Legislation

A system to provide citizens with access to health insurance through a combination of private and public plans. Several key provisions: the creation of the Commonwealth Health Insurance Connector Authority; the establishment of the subsidized Commonwealth Care Health Insurance Programme (C-CHIP); the employer Fair Share Contribution; and a mandate that each individual have insurance. The statute also expands MassHealth (Medicaid and SCHIP) coverage for children and restores MassHealth benefits like dental care and eyeglasses. A merger of the individual (non-group) insurance market into the small group market will allow individuals to get lower group insurance rates. Payment rates are increased to hospitals and physicians, and a new "Quality and Cost Council," will issue quality standards and publicize provider performance.

Commonwealth Health Insurance Connector Authority

The Connector is designed as a clearinghouse for insurance plans and payments. It performs the following functions:

— It runs the Commonwealth Care programme for low-income residents (below 300% of the poverty level) who do not qualify for MassHealth.

— It offers health insurance plans for individuals who:

- are not working
- are employed by a small business (less than 50 employees) that uses the Connector to offer health insurance. These residents will purchase insurance with pre-tax income.
- are not qualified under their large employer plan
- are self-employed, part-time workers, or work for multiple employers

— It sets premium subsidy levels for Commonwealth Care.

— It defines "affordability" for purposes of the individual mandate

The Connector is run by the Commonwealth Health Insurance Connector Authority, an independent agency with a 10-member board. The Connector will make health insurance portable by allowing employees to keep the same plan even if they leave an employer. The Connector will also allow employees to aggregate the contributions of multiple employers, e.g. if they are part-time workers or work for multiple employers, and apply them to one insurance plan.

Commonwealth Care Health Insurance Programme

Commonwealth Care will provide a subsidized private insurance health plan for individuals without health insurance. Commonwealth Care will cover those not qualified for MassHealth below 300% of the federal poverty level. No deductibles may be imposed. For individuals below the poverty line, no premiums will be charged. For those above the poverty level, a sliding scale premium schedule based on income is used to determine the amount of money a person contributes to their policy. Commonwealth Care for those below poverty will be available through the Connector, starting October 1, 2006. Plans for those between 100% and 300% of the poverty line will begin on January 1, 2007.

Fair Share Contribution

Employers with more than ten employees must offer provide a "fair and reasonable contribution" to the premium of health insurance for employees. Employers who do not will be assessed an annual fair share contribution that will not exceed $295 per employee per year. The fair share contribution will be paid into the Commonwealth Care Trust Fund to fund Commonwealth Care. The Division of Health Care Finance and Policy will define what contribution level meets the "fair and reasonable" test in the statute. There is an additional Free Rider Surcharge that can be assessed to the employer. This surcharge is different from the fair share contribution. The surcharge is applied when an employer does not arrange for health insurance, such as by setting up a payroll deduction system, and has employees who receive care that is paid from the uncompensated care pool. If an employee receives free care more than three times or all of an employer's employees use free care a total of five times, then the employer must pay a portion of the health care costs.

Individual Insurance Requirement

Residents of Massachusetts must have health insurance coverage. Residents must indicate on their tax forms for the 2007 tax year if they have insurance, have a waiver for religious reasons, or have a waiver from the Connector. The Connector waiver can be obtained if the resident demonstrates that there is no Connector plan that is affordable. If a resident does not have coverage and does not have a waiver, the Department of Revenue will enforce the insurance requirement. In 2007, the penalty will be the loss of the personal exemption. In future tax years the individual must pay for half the cost of the lowest available yearly premium which will be enforced as an assessed addition to the individual's income tax.

Implementation

The implementation began in June, 2006, with the appointment of members of the Connector board, and the naming of Jon Kingsdale, a Tufts Health Plan official, as executive director of the Connector. The Board started meeting biweekly. On July 1, MassHealth began covering dental care and other benefits, and began enrolling children between 200% and 300% of the poverty level.

The federal Centers for Medicare and Medicaid Services approved the state's waiver application on July 26, 2006, allowing the state to begin enrolling 10,500 from the waitlist for the MassHealth Essential programme, which provides Medicaid coverage to long-term unemployed adults below the poverty line.

In September, 2006, the Division of Health Care Finance

and Policy issued regulations defining "fair and reasonable" for the fair share assessment. The regulations provide that companies with 11 or more full-time equivalent employees will meet the "fair and reasonable" test if at least 25 percent of those employees are enrolled in that firm's health plan and the company is making a contribution toward it. A business that fails that test may still be deemed to offer a "fair and reasonable" contribution if the company offers to pay at least 33 percent of an individual's health insurance premium.

Also in September, the Connector Board set premium levels and copayments for Commonwealth Care plans. Premiums will vary from $18 per month, for individuals with incomes 100%-150% of the poverty line, to $106 per month for individuals with incomes 250%-300% of poverty. The Connector approved two copayment schemes for plans for people 200%-300% of poverty. One plan will have higher premiums and lower copayments, while a second choice will have lower premiums and higher copayments.

Litigation

The possibility exists that a legal challenge to the law may arise under the presumption that it is an attempt to preempt the federal Employee Retirement Income Security Act (ERISA). A somewhat similar law with respect to employer spending on health insurance in Maryland was struck down by a federal judge on July 19, 2006. The law in question had required employers with more than 10,000 employees to spend no less than 8% of their payroll on health insurance benefits. The ruling effectively delineated that states cannot interfere in the administration of employer provided benefits to their employees and such interference was a violation of federal law.

8

Public Health Acts, Guidelines and Ethics

PART I: ADMINISTRATION OF THE GOVERNMENT

PUBLIC HEALTH

Dispensaries

Section 51. Hospitals, Institutions for Unwed Mothers, or Clinics; Licensing

Section 51. The department shall issue for a term of two years, and shall renew for like terms, a license, subject to revocation by it for cause, to any person, city, town, or county it deems responsible and suitable to establish or maintain a hospital, an institution for the care of unwed mothers or a clinic, which meets the requirements of the department established in accordance with its rules and regulations. In the case of the transfer of ownership of a hospital, an institution for the care of unwed mothers or a clinic, the application of the new owner for a license, when filed with the department on the date of transfer of ownership, shall have the effect of a license for a period of three months. If a license has not been issued by the department upon the expiration of said three months period, all the patients shall be transferred or discharged from such hospital or such institution for unwed mothers, and the hospital, institution for unwed mothers, or clinic, as the case may be, shall cease operating.

No original license shall be issued to establish or maintain a hospital, an institution for the care of unwed mothers or a clinic providing ambulatory surgery as defined by section twenty-five B, unless there is determination by the department that there is need for such a facility at the designated location; provided, however, that no such determination shall be required with respect to original licensure of any hospital or clinic which, pursuant to the provisions of section twenty-five C1/2, is exempt from the provisions of section twenty-five C; and provided further, that no license shall be issued or renewed to any applicant to establish or maintain an acute hospital as defined, if the department has been notified by the division of health care policy and finance that such applicant or such hospital owes an outstanding obligation to the Uncompensated Care Trust Fund pursuant to section 18.

Each hospital shall give the department an annual written statement containing a licensure adjustment calculated pursuant to this section as of the first day of such hospital's fiscal year, and the department shall adjust the hospital's total licensed bed capacity accordingly. As of such date, each hospital's number of licensed acute-care medical-surgical beds, excluding all critical care beds, shall be adjusted to equal the lesser of: (a) the number of such licensed beds as reported for the prior year on division of health care finance and policy form 403, schedule III, column 4, line 1; or (b) a number equal to the average daily census for such prior year divided by seventy-five hundredths; provided, however, that no such adjustment shall be made on or after October first, nineteen hundred and ninety-three, if such adjustment would result in the loss of the hospital's eligibility for an additional payment amount pursuant to section 1886 (d) (5) (F) of the Social Security Act if at any time during the prior fiscal year said hospital serves a disproportionate number of low income patients as defined in section 1886 (d) (5) (F) (v) of said Social Security Act. Such average daily census shall be calculated by dividing the number reported in division of health care finance and policy form 403, schedule III, column 6, line 1, by three hundred and sixty-five. If a hospital experiences eighty-five per cent average occupancy for its adult medical-surgical beds excluding all critical care beds for three consecutive months, it may, by letter application documenting such occupancy, increase its licensed number of such beds to a number equal to the average daily census of adult medical-surgical beds excluding all critical care beds, divided by seventy-five hundredths, or to a number equal to its number of licensed beds for the preceding fiscal year, whichever is less. The department shall approve or disapprove such application within ten days after filing, on the basis of a review limited to the sole issue of whether such hospital is in fact experiencing such occupancy. If such application has not been acted upon by the department within such time limit, the application shall be deemed approved. Notwithstanding the foregoing, the department may permit a hospital to increase its licensed bed capacity by the number of beds for which such hospital qualifies according to a determination of need by the department pursuant to sections twenty-five B to twenty-five G, inclusive and provided further, that the department may retrospectively and prospectively waive the automatic bed delicensure provisions imposed pursuant to this paragraph to assist financially troubled hospitals for the purpose of qualifying for medicare disproportionate share reimbursement, and for other reasonable purposes.

Each licensee shall maintain its licensed bed capacity at all times in accordance with the provisions of this chapter and all applicable rules and regulations promulgated by the department.

No original license shall be issued to establish a hospital, except a college and school infirmary, unless it complies with the construction standards of the state building code and is of at least type 1-B fireproof construction.

In the case of new construction of a hospital, an institution for unwed mothers or a clinic, or in the case of alterations or additions to an existing hospital, an institution for unwed mothers or a clinic, preliminary architectural plans and final architectural plans and specifications shall be submitted to the division of hospital facilities of the department. Written approval of the final architectural plans and specifications shall be obtained from said division prior to said new construction or alterations or additions.

No original license shall be issued nor shall a license be renewed hereunder unless there shall be first submitted to the department by the authorities in charge of the hospital, the institution for unwed mothers or the clinic, with respect to each building occupied by patients, (1) a certificate of inspection of the egresses, the means of preventing the spread of fire and the apparatus for extinguishing fire, issued by an inspector of the division of inspection of the department of public safety, and (2) a certificate of inspection issued by the head of the local fire department certifying compliance with the local ordinances.

Any applicant for an original or renewal license who is aggrieved by a written disapproval of a certificate of inspection by the head of the local fire department or by the division of inspection of the department of public safety, may, within thirty days from such disapproval, appeal in writing, to the department of public safety. Failure to either approve or disapprove within thirty days, after a written request by an applicant, shall be deemed a disapproval.

If the department of public safety approves the issuance of a certificate of inspection, it shall forthwith be issued by the agency that failed to approve. If said department disapproves, the applicant may appeal therefrom to the superior court. Failure of the department of public safety to either approve or disapprove the issuance of a certificate of inspection within thirty days after receipt of an appeal shall be deemed a disapproval. No original license shall be issued and no license shall be renewed by the department of public health until issuance of an approved certificate of inspection, as required in this section.

Upon a written request by an applicant who is aggrieved by the revocation of a license or the refusal of the department to renew a license, the commissioner and the council shall hold a public hearing, after due notice, and thereafter they may modify, affirm or reverse the action of the department. In no case shall the revocation of such a license take effect in less than thirty days after written notification by the department to the hospital, the institution for unwed mothers or the clinic. There shall be no new admissions to such hospital, an institution for unwed mothers or a clinic during the thirty day period herein referred to; and upon the expiration of said thirty days all the patients shall be transferred or discharged therefrom and the hospital or the institution for unwed mothers or the clinic shall cease operating.

The fee for the issue or renewal of each license shall be determined annually by the commissioner of administration under the provision of section three B, for a hospital or an institution for unwed mothers and for all clinics. The license shall not be transferable and shall be issued only for the premises described in the application.

No hospital licensed pursuant to this section shall permit

early discharge, defined as less than forty-eight hours for a vaginal delivery and ninety-six hours for a caesarean delivery except in accordance with rules and regulations established by the department of public health.

The department of public health shall promulgate rules and regulations as required under section seventeen C, section ten A, section forty-seven F, section eight H and section four H; provided, however, that the standards shall be consistent with the most current guidelines established by the American College of Obstetricians and Gynecologists and the American Academy of Pediatrics.

PUBLIC HEALTH LAW, ETHICS, AND HUMAN RIGHTS: MAPPING THE ISSUES

This *Reader* offers an organised selection of government reports, scholarly articles, and court cases on public health law, ethics, and human rights. The publication of a *Reader* on these subjects may suggest that a coherent, systematic understanding of the relationships between public health law, ethics, and human rights exists. Despite the deep traditions in these separate fields, they have rarely cross-fertilized. For the most part, each of these fields has adopted its own terminologies and forms of reasoning. To the extent that scholars in law, ethics, or human rights have engaged in sustained examinations of issues in health, they have written principally about medical care. This introductory chapter maps the important features of, and issues in, these respective fields as they pertain to the theory and practice of public health. Part I of the Reader explores public health, ethics, and human rights in more detail. Part II examines major issues in public health law, including constitutional, administrative, and tort law. Part III focuses on some of the major controversies and tradeoffs involved in public health theory and practice. And Part IV conceptualizes a vision for public health in a new century.

I. Public Health

In thinking about the application of ethical or human rights to problems in public health, it is important first to understand what we mean by public health. How is the field defined and what is its content—its mission, functions, and services? Who engages in the practice of public health—government, the private sector, charities, community-based organisations? What are the principal methods or techniques of public health practitioners? In truth, finding answers to these fundamental questions is not easy because the field of public health is highly eclectic and conflicted (Beaglehole and Bonita 1997). For a summary of the definition, mission, functions, and jurisdiction of public health.

Definitions of public health vary widely, ranging from the utopian conception of the World Health Organisation of an ideal state of physical and mental health to a more concrete listing of public health practices. Charles-Edward A. Winslow (1920, 30), for example, defined public health as "the science and the art of preventing disease, prolonging life, and promoting physical health and efficiency through organised community efforts for the sanitation of the environment, the control of community infections, the education of the individual in principles of personal hygiene, [and] the organisation of medical and nursing service for the early diagnosis and preventive treatment of disease." More recent definitions focus on "positive health," emphasizing a person's complete well-being (*Lancet* Editorial 1997, 229). Definitions of positive health include at least four constructs: a healthy body, high-quality personal relationships, a sense of purpose in life, and self-regard and resilience (Rowe and Kahn 1998).

The Institute of Medicine (IOM) (1988, 19), in its seminal report on the *Future of Public Health*, proposed one of the most influential contemporary definitions: "Public health is what we, as a society, do collectively to assure the conditions for people to be healthy."

The IOM's definition can be appreciated by examining its constituent parts. The emphasis on cooperative and mutually shared obligation ("we, as a society") reinforces that collective entities (e.g., governments and communities) take responsibility for healthy populations. Individuals can do a great deal to safeguard their health, particularly if they have the economic means to do so. They can purchase housing, clothing, food, and medical care. Each person can also behave in ways that promote health and safety by eating healthy foods, exercising, using safety equipment (e.g., seatbelts and motorcycle helmets), or refraining from smoking, using illicit drugs, or drinking alcoholic beverages excessively. Yet, there is a great deal that individuals cannot do to secure their health and, therefore, these individuals need to organise, build together, and share resources. Acting alone, people cannot achieve environmental protection, hygiene and sanitation, clean air and surface water, uncontaminated food and drinking water, safe roads and products, and control of infectious disease. Each of these collective goods, and many more, are achievable only by organised and sustained community activities (Gostin 2000a).

The IOM definition also makes clear that even the most organised and socially conscious society cannot guarantee complete physical and mental well-being. There will always be a certain amount of injury and disease in the population that is beyond the reach of individuals or government. The role of public health, therefore, is to "assure the *conditions* for people to be healthy." These conditions include a variety of educational, economic, social, and environmental factors that are necessary for good health.

Most definitions share the premise that the subject of

public health is the health of populations—rather than the health of individuals—and that this goal is reached by a generally high level of health throughout society, rather than the best possible health for a few. The field of public health is concerned with health promotion and disease prevention throughout society. Consequently, public health is less interested in clinical interactions between health care professionals and patients, and more interested in devising broad strategies to prevent, or ameliorate, injury, and disease.

Scholars and practitioners are conflicted about the "reach" or domain of public health. Some prefer a narrow focus on the proximal risk factors for injury and disease. The role of public health agencies, according to this perspective, is to identify risks or harms and intervene to prevent or ameliorate them. This has been the traditional role of public health, exercising discrete powers such as surveillance (e.g., screening and reporting), injury prevention (e.g., safe consumer products), and infectious disease control (e.g., vaccination, partner notification, and quarantine).

Others prefer a broad focus on the sociocultural foundations of health. Those favouring this position see public health as an all-embracing enterprise bonded by the common value of societal wellbeing. They claim that the jurisdiction of public health reaches "social ills rooted in distal social structures." (Meyer and Schwartz 2000). Ultimately, the field is interested in the equitable distribution of social and economic resources because social status, race, and wealth are important influences on the health of populations (Marmot and Wilkinson 1999). This inclusive direction for public health is gaining popularity; many of the government's health objectives for 2010 seek reductions in health disparities. The determinants of health according to Department of Health and Human Services (2000)—

physical environment, behaviour and biology, and social environment. Using this vision, public health researchers and practitioners have ventured into areas of general social policy including violence, war, homelessness, and discrimination (Breakey 1997).

The expansive view of public health may well be justified by the importance of culture, poverty, and powerlessness on the health of populations. Yet, to many, this all-embracing notion is troublesome. First, there is the problem of excessive breadth. Almost everything human beings undertake impacts the population's health, but that does not justify an overly-inclusive definition of public health. The field of public health appears less credible if it appears to overreach.

Second, there is the problem of expertise. Admittedly, the public health professions incorporate a wide variety of disciplines (e.g., occupational health, health education, epidemiology, and nursing) with different skills and functions. But public health professionals do not possess all the skills necessary to intervene on behavioural, social, physical, and environmental levels (e.g., competence in behaviour sciences, economics, and engineering).

Finally, there is the problem of political and public support. By espousing controversial issues of economic redistribution and social restructuring, the field risks losing its legitimacy. Public health gains credibility from its adherence to science, and if the field strays too far into political advocacy, it may lose the appearance of objectivity.

If public health has such a broad meaning, then who engages in the work of public health—government, the private sector, academia, charities, community-based organisations? At the governmental level, public health has a significant jurisdictional problem. Even the most powerful public health agency cannot exercise direct authority over the full range of activities that affect health. Many of the determinants of health are normally the province of other agencies (e.g., agencies concerned with education, agriculture, transportation, housing, child welfare, and criminal justice). Furthermore, much of the behaviour that public health authorities try to change (e.g., exercise and diet) is not subject to direct legal regulation at all. At the same time, many of the institutions that affect the public's health are not within government, such as managed care organisations, business and labor, community-based groups, and academic institutions (Gostin, Burris, and Lazzarini 1999; Bowser and Gostin 1999). Thus, scholars need to consider the actors who carry out the work of public health. It matters a great deal in law and ethics to understand who is acting, with what authority, and with what resources. For example, society is prepared to allow government to wield powers to coerce (e.g., tax, inspect, license, and quarantine) that would be unacceptable in the private sector.

What are the principal methodologies of public health practitioners? Because of the field's broad sweep, the techniques of public health are highly diverse (Sommer and Akhter 2000). For example, public health practitioners monitor health status, calling for skills in epidemiology and biostatistics; inform and educate the public, calling for skills in education and communication; and create health policy and enforce law, calling for skills in leadership and politics. This description does not account for the many subjects in the field of public health requiring expertise in domains such as infectious diseases (e.g., virology and bacteriology), the environment (e.g., toxicology), and injuries (e.g., behavioural and social sciences). As the IOM (1988) observed: "public health's subject matter. . . necessitate[s] the involvement of a broad spectrum of professional disciplines. In fact, . . . public health is a coalition of professions united by their shared mission."

The field of public health is caught in a dilemma. If it conceives itself too narrowly then public health will be accused of lacking vision. It will fail to see the root causes of ill health and fail to utilize a broad range of social, economic, and behavioural tools necessary to achieve healthier populations (McGinnis and Foege 1993). At the same time, if it conceives itself too expansively then public health will be accused of overreaching and invading a sphere reserved for politics, not science. It will lose the ability to explain its mission and functions in comprehensible terms and, consequently, to sell public health in the marketplace of politics and priorities (Burris 1997b).

II. Public Health Law

As we have just seen, the question "What is Public Health?" is much more difficult than it first appears. Despite the lack of conceptual clarity, it is important to study carefully the legal foundations of public health, its ethical dimensions, and its relationship to human rights.

The preservation of the public health is among the most important goals of government. The enactment and enforcement of law, moreover, is a primary means with which government creates the conditions for people to lead healthier and safer lives. Law creates a mission for public health authorities, assigns their functions, and specifies the manner in which they may exercise their authority (Gostin, Burris, and Lazzarini 1999). The law is a tool in public health work which is used to influence norms for healthy behaviour, identify and respond to health threats, and set and enforce health and safety standards. The most important social debates about public health take place in legal fora—legislatures, courts, and administrative agencies—

and in the law's language of rights, duties, and justice. It is no exaggeration to say that "the field of public health . . . could not long exist in the manner in which we know it today except for its sound legal basis" (Grad 1990, 4).

Despite its importance, there is a scarcity of legal scholarship relating to public health. In the companion text I define public health law as "The study of the legal powers and duties of the state to assure the conditions for people to be healthy and the limits on that power to constrain the autonomy, privacy, liberty, proprietary, or other legally protected interests of individuals for protection or promotion of community health." Five characteristics help distinguish public health law from the vast literature on law and medicine (1) the role of *government* in advancing the public's health; (2) the *population-based* perspective; (3) the *relationship* between the people and the state; (4) the *services* and scientific methodologies; and (5) the role of *coercion*.

Public health law scholars, therefore, are interested in government authority to prevent injury and disease and to promote the public's health, as well as in the constraints on state action to protect individual freedom. Government has ample authority to act for the common good but also must exercise that power within the constraints of the Constitution.

Law can be an effective tool to achieve the goal of improved health for the population. Law, regulation, and litigation, like other public health prevention strategies, intervene at a variety of levels, each designed to secure safer and healthier populations. First, government interventions are aimed at *individual* behaviour through education (e.g., health communication campaigns), incentives (e.g., taxing and spending powers), or deterrence (e.g., civil and criminal penalties for risky behaviours). Second, the law regulates the *agents of behaviour change* by requiring safer product design (e.g., safety standards and indirect regulation through the tort system). Finally, the law alters the informational (e.g., advertising restraints), physical (e.g., city planning and housing codes), or business (e.g., inspections and licenses) *environments*.

Government engages in the work of public health through three separate branches— legislative, executive, and judicial. The Constitution provides a system of checks and balances where no single branch of government can act without some degree of oversight and control by another. Separation of powers is essential to public health, for each branch of government possesses a unique constitutional authority: (1) legislatures create health policy and allocate the resources necessary to effectuate it; (2) executive agencies implement health policy, promulgate health regulations, and enforce regulatory standards; and (3) courts interpret law and resolve legal disputes. As a society, we forego the possibility of bold public health governance by any given branch in exchange for constitutional checks and balances that prevent government overreaching and assure political accountability.

Public health law is concerned with the tradeoffs entailed in the exercise of government power. Under what circumstances should government be permitted to act to achieve a public good when the consequence of that act is to invade a sphere of individual liberty? This is the kind of question that intrigues scholars interested in law and the public's health. Rather than using ethical discourse to resolve these conflicts, the law uses the language of duties, powers, and rights.

It is clear from the foregoing description that public health law is a vast field incorporating thinking in a variety of legal subspecialties—constitutional, civil, administrative, and tort law. The Constitution affords the federal government certain powers and limits the authority of all governments to protect a sphere of freedom. Civil and administrative law is concerned with the body of statutes and regulations that set health and safety standards, together with agency powers to interpret and enforce those standards. Tort law provides a method of indirect regulation through the courts. By levying damages for certain kinds of harm, tort law can provide powerful disincentives to risk behaviours (e.g., litigation against cigarette and firearm manufacturers). As the chapters in this *Reader* unfold, these legal dimensions are explored (see Part II).

III. Public Health Ethics

The field of bioethics has richly informed the practice of medicine and decisions about the allocation of health care resources. Bioethicists, at least until recently, have not devoted the same sustained attention to problems in public health (Steinbock and Beauchamp 1999; Bradely and Burls 2000; Coughlin and Beauchamp 1996). A critical unanswered question is whether public health ethics have features which are distinct from conventional bioethics. Are ethical principles, or the methods of ethical analysis, materially different when applied to populations than when applied to individual patients? In thinking about this question it will be helpful to consider public health ethics from at least two perspectives: the ethics *of* public health professionals (professional ethics) and ethics *in* public health theory and practice (applied ethics).

The ethics of public health are concerned with the ethical dimensions of professionalism and the moral trust that society bestows on public health professionals to act for the common welfare (Callahan 2000). This form of ethical discourse stresses the distinct history and traditions of the profession, seeking to create a culture of professionalism among public health students and practitioners. It instills in professionals a sense of public duty and trust. Professional ethics are role oriented, helping practitioners to act in virtuous ways as they undertake their functions.

Many professional groups such as physicians and attorneys hold themselves accountable through a set of ethical guidelines, but public health professionals have no code of ethics. Perhaps the explanation is that no single public health profession exists, but rather a variety of different disciplines. Indeed, some public health disciplines have their own ethical codes—e.g., epidemiologists and public health educators. Nevertheless, a code of ethics, or at least a well-articulated values statement, could increase the status of the field and help clarify the distinctive ethical dilemmas faced by public health professionals. Public health professionals work in a field of considerable moral ambiguity where guidance could be instructive.

A public health code of ethics would have to confront the salient issue of fiduciary responsibility. To whom do public health professionals owe a duty of loyalty and how can these professionals know what actions are morally acceptable? Physicians, attorneys, and accountants have a fiduciary duty to their clients that informs their moral world. For example, client-centered professions usually adhere to the principle that the professional serves the client, advises the client fully and honestly, takes instructions from the client, and avoids acting against the client's best interests.

In the context of public health, the community might be regarded as the "client." The problem is that it is unclear what constitutes a "community"— the notion is often vague and fragmented. In any given situation, different groups may claim to represent community interests. If the community's wants and needs are not easily ascertained, should public health professionals make their own judgments about communal interests? Public health professionals may, at times, coerce some members of the community, not necessarily in the community's best interests, but in the interests of others. When thinking about public health's complex relationship to populations, is the concept of fiduciary duty helpful as an ethical value?

Do public health professionals have a duty to tell the full truth and, if so, under what standard should they be judged? Public health professionals may earnestly believe that their mission requires vigorous interventions to prevent risk behaviours (e.g., smoking) or encourage health-promoting behaviours (e.g., screening and treatment). To achieve these beneficent objectives, public health professionals may exaggerate the risks or benefits or make claims that are insufficiently grounded in science (Wikler and Beauchamp 1995). Suppose public health professionals know that the risk of sexual transmission of HIV in middle class, low prevalence areas is relatively low. Are they obliged to disclose this fact when advising men to wear condoms? How would an ethical code address the nuanced question of "truth telling" by public health professionals?

A second form of public health ethics might be called ethics *in* public health theory and practice. Ethics in public health is concerned not so much with the character of professionals as with the ethical dimensions of the public health enterprise itself. Here, scholars study the philosophical knowledge and analytic reasoning necessary for careful thinking and decision making in creating and implementing public health policy. This kind of "applied" ethics is situation or case oriented, seeking to understand morally appropriate decisions in concrete cases. Scholars can helpfully apply general ethical theory and detached analytical reasoning to the societal debates common in public health.

The application of general ethical principles to public health decisions can be difficult and complicated. Since the mission of public health is to achieve the greatest health benefits for the greatest number of people, it draws from the traditions of utilitarianism or consequentialism. The "public health model," argue Buchanan (2000) and his colleagues, uncritically assumes that the appropriate mode of evaluating options is some form of cost-benefit (or cost-effectiveness) calculation— the aggregation of goods and bads (costs and benefits) across individuals. Public health, according to this view, appears to permit, or even require, that the most fundamental interests of individuals be sacrificed in order to produce the best overall outcome.

This characterisation misperceives, or at least oversimplifies, the public health approach. The field of public health is interested in securing the greatest benefits for the most people. But public health does not simply aggregate benefits and burdens, choosing the policy that produces the most good and the least harm. Rather, the overwhelming majority of public health interventions are intended to benefit the whole population, without knowingly harming individuals or groups. When public health authorities work in the areas of tobacco control, the environment, or occupational safety, for example, their belief is that everyone will benefit from smoking cessation, clean air, and safe workplaces. Certainly, public health focuses almost exclusively on one vision of the "common good" (health, not wealth or prosperity), but this is not the same thing as sacrificing fundamental interests to produce the best overall outcome.

The public health approach, of course, does follow a version of the harm principle. Thus, public health authorities regulate individuals or businesses that endanger the community. The objective is to prevent unreasonable risks that jeopardize the public's health and safety— e.g, polluting a stream, practicing medicine without a license, or exposing others to an infectious disease. More controversially, public health authorities often recommend paternalistic interventions such as mandatory seat belt or motorcycle helmet laws. Public health authorities reason that the sacrifice asked of individuals is relatively minimal and the communal benefits substantial. Few public health experts advocate denial of fundamental interests in the name of paternalism. In the public health model, individual interests in autonomy, privacy, liberty, and property are taken seriously, but they do not invariably trump community health benefits. The public health approach, therefore, differs from modern liberalism primarily in its preferences for balancing— public health favours community benefits, while liberalism favours liberty interests. Characterizing public health as a utilitarian sacrifice of fundamental personal interests is as unfair as characterizing liberalism as a sacrifice of vital communal interests. Both traditions would deny this kind of oversimplification.

Scholars in bioethics have demonstrated convincingly the power and importance of individual freedom. However, they have given insufficient attention to equally strong values of partnership, citizenship, and community (Beauchamp 1998). As members of a society in which we all share a common bond, we also have an obligation to protect and defend the community against threats to health, safety, and security. Members of society owe a duty—one to another—to promote the common good. A new public health ethic should advance the idea that individuals benefit from being part of a well-regulated society that reduces risks that all members share.

There remains much work to do in public health ethics.

What is the moral standing that should be attached to the collective good? Does the health of the community have a moral standing that is independent of the health of individuals within that population? Under what circumstances should individual interests yield to achieve an aggregate benefit for the population?

At the same time, ethics in public health raise the important issue of social justice. How can society equitably allocate benefits or services, on the one hand, and burdens or costs, on the other? Does an otherwise effective policy become unfair if it disproportionately disadvantages a racial, ethnic, or religious group? For example, public health professionals often advocate primary enforcement of seatbelt laws so police can stop a driver simply for failure to comply with the law. But what if primary seatbelt laws are enforced disproportionately against African Americans? Similarly, agencies advocate an increase in the cigarette tax, knowing that the tax is highly regressive. Is it fair to disproportionately burden the poor who use tobacco products to achieve generally lower levels of smoking in the population?

Public health professionals routinely face these and many other kinds of dilemmas that could be informed by ethics scholarship. Think about the dilemmas that occur in the everyday practice of public health. When do educational messages cross the line to become persuasion or propaganda? When does surveillance or research unacceptably interfere with privacy? Under what circumstances— consistent with free expression— can agencies restrict commercial advertising? In regulating professionals and businesses (e.g., licenses, inspections, and nuisance abatements), how much deference should agencies give to property interests?

In addition to "professional" and "applied" ethics, it is possible to think of an "advocacy" ethic informed by the single overriding value of a healthy community (Jennings 2000). Under this rationale, public health authorities think they know what is ethically appropriate and their function is to advocate for that social goal. This populist ethic serves the interests of populations, particularly the powerless and oppressed, and its methods are principally pragmatic and political. Public health professionals strive to convince the public and its representative political bodies that healthy populations and reduced inequalities are the preferred social responses.

Public health ethics, therefore, can illuminate the field of public health in several ways. Ethics can offer guidance on (i) the meaning of public health professionalism and the ethical practice of the profession; (ii) the moral weight and value of the community's health and wellbeing; (iii) the recurring themes of the field and the dilemmas faced in everyday public health practice; and (iv) the role of advocacy to achieve the goal of safer and healthier populations.

IV. Human Rights

The language of human rights is used in different, but overlapping, ways. Some use human rights language to mean a set of entitlements under international law, others use human rights to mean a set of ethical standards that stress the paramount importance of individuals, and still others use human rights for its aspirational, or rhetorical, qualities. A scholar is bound to be concerned when the terminology of human rights is invoked without clarifying the sense in which it is intended.

Legal scholars and practitioners use human rights to refer to a body of international law that originated in response to the egregious affronts to peace and human dignity committed during World War II. The main source of human rights law within the United Nations system is the

International Bill of Human Rights comprising the United Nations Charter, the Universal Declaration of Human Rights (UDHR), and two International Covenants of Human Rights. Human rights are also protected under regional systems, including those in American, European, African, and Arab countries.

In its preamble, the United Nations Charter articulates the international community's determination "to reaffirm faith in fundamental human rights, [and] in the dignity and worth of the human person." The Charter, as a binding treaty, pledges member states to promote universal respect for, and observance of, human rights and fundamental freedoms for all without distinction as to race, sex, language, or religion (arts. 55–56).

The UDHR, adopted in 1948, built upon the promise of the Charter by identifying specific rights and freedoms that deserve promotion and protection. The UDHR was the organised international community's first attempt to establish "a common standard of achievement for all peoples and all nations" to promote human rights (Preamble). The UDHR has largely fulfilled the promise of its preamble, becoming the "common standard" for evaluating respect for human rights. Although it was not promulgated to legally bind member states, its key provisions have so often been applied and accepted that they are now widely considered to have attained the status of customary international law.

The adoption of the UDHR set the stage for a binding, treaty-based scheme to promote and protect human rights. The International Covenant on Civil and Political Rights (ICCPR) and the International Covenant on Economic, Social and Cultural Rights (ICESCR) were adopted in 1966 and entered into force in 1976. The United States has ratified the ICCPR but not the ICESCR. The rights contained in the ICCPR are principally negative or defensive in character, affording individuals a sphere of protection from government restraint. These rights, which are to be respected without discrimination, include the following: the right to life, liberty, and security of person; the prohibition of slavery, torture, and cruel, inhuman, or degrading treatment; the right to an effective judicial remedy; the prohibition of arbitrary arrest, detention, and exile; freedom from arbitrary interference with privacy, family, or home; freedom of movement; freedom of conscience, religion, expression, and association; and the right to participate in government.

The UDHR characterizes economic, social, and cultural rights as “indispensable for [a person’s] dignity and the development of his personality” (art. 22). The ICESCR forms the foundation for “positive rights,” that is, those requiring affirmative duties of the state to provide services. Such positive rights include the right to social security, the right to education, the right to work, the right to receive equal pay for equal work and to remuneration ensuring “an existence worthy of human dignity,” and the right to share in the cultural life of the community and “to share in scientific advancement and its benefits” (arts. 22–27). Article 12 of the ICESCR requires governments to recognize “the right of everyone to the highest attainable standard of physical and mental health.” Article 25 of the UDHR also expressly recognizes a right to health:

Everyone has the right to a standard of living adequate for the health and well-being of himself and his family, including food, clothing, housing and medical care and necessary social services, and the right to security in the event of unemployment, sickness, disability, widowhood, old age or other lack of livelihood in circumstances beyond his control.

The two Covenants diverge in their treatment of permissible limitations. The ICCPR recognizes that certain rights are so fundamental as to be absolute and proscribes any derogation of them. Nonderogable rights include the right to life (art. 6); freedom from torture and from cruel, inhuman, or degrading treatment or punishment (art. 7); the right to recognition as a person before the law (art. 16); and freedom of thought, conscience, and religion (art. 18). The ICCPR states that other rights may be justifiably limited under certain conditions. Freedom of movement, for example, may be justifiably limited where restrictions are "provided for by law, are necessary to protect national security, public order, public health or morals or the rights and freedoms of others. . . " (art. 12.3). The ICESCR, on the other hand, permits "such limitations as are determined by law only in so far as this may be compatible with the nature of these rights and solely for the purpose of promoting the general welfare in a democratic society." (art. 4).

Human rights law follows a set of internationally agreed rules specified in the text of treaties and other instruments, is informed by precedent, and is interpreted by tribunals and commissions. International human rights law seldom provides easy answers, but struggles to define and enforce human rights in the context of the legitimate powers of governments and the needs of communities.

Ethicists use the language of human rights for related, but different, purposes. The fields of ethics and human rights share an abiding belief in the paramount importance of individual rights and interests, but beyond that their perspectives diverge. While human rights scholars stress the importance of treaty obligations, ethicists seldom refer to international law doctrine. While human rights scholars rely on text and precedent, ethicists employ philosophical reasoning and argumentation. When ethicists adopt the language of international human rights, there is bound to be a certain amount of confusion. For example, if ethicists claim that health care is a "human right," do they mean that a definable and enforceable right under international law exists or simply that philosophical principles such as justice support this claim?

Finally, public health students, as well as the lay public, often use the language of human rights for its aspirational, or rhetorical, qualities. Major public health schools, such as the Johns Hopkins University and Harvard University, give their students a copy of the UDHR at commencement or offer special certificates in human rights. When "rights" language is invoked, it is intended to convey the fundamental importance of the claim. It expresses the idea that government should adhere to certain standards, or provide certain services, because it is right and just to do so. Human rights as a symbol commands reverence and respect. Used in this aspirational sense, human rights need not be supported by text, precedent, or reasoning; they are self-evident and government's responsibility simply is to conform.

Human rights, then, have features in common with ethics, but they are different fields. Human rights, like ethics, are often concerned with individual rights and interests, and, like advocacy ethics, human rights convey a sense of moral certainty. However, international human rights are also quite distinct from ethics. The field of human rights is based on a body of rules and precedents which are intended to express binding duties. It is complex and evolving, usually rejecting easy resolutions to the conflict between individual interests and collective goods.

The field of human rights has much work to do if it is to contribute usefully to health policy analysis. For example, human rights scholars and advocates have not clarified the meaning of the right to health (Gostin and Lazzarini 1997; Jamar 1994). The conceptualisation of health as a human right, and not simply a moral claim, suggests that states possess binding obligations to respect, defend, and promote that entitlement (Leary 1994). Considerable disagreement, however, exists as to whether "health" is a meaningful, identifiable, operational, and enforceable right, or whether it is merely aspirational or rhetorical. A right to health that is too broadly defined lacks clear content and is less likely to have a meaningful effect. If health is, in WHO's words, truly "a state of complete physical, mental and social well-being," then it can never be achieved. Even if this definition were construed as a reasonable, as opposed to an absolute, standard, it remains difficult to implement, and is unlikely to be justiciable. Vast scholarship and litigation in international fora were required to define and enforce civil and political rights. However, social and economic rights, notably the right to health, deserve the same rigorous and sustained attention (Gostin 2000c). This is beginning to happen in international fora (Toebes 1999b). For example, the United Nations Committee on Economic, Social, and Cultural Rights recently offered detailed guidance on the meaning of the right to health

9

Competition Laws for Hospitals, Physicians and Pharmaceutical

COMPETITION LAW: HOSPITALS

I. Introduction

Analyses of the likely competitive effects of hospital mergers have been an important part of antitrust enforcement since the FTC issued its first hospital merger complaint in 1981.Most hospital mergers and acquisitions do not present competitive concerns. The *Department of Justice and Federal Trade Commission Statements of Antitrust Enforcement Policy in Health Care (Health Care Statements)* specifically set forth a safety zone for hospital mergers that will be rarely (if ever) challenged by the Agencies. Indeed, since 1981, the Commission and DOJ have challenged relatively few hospital mergers, in some instances seeking relief only for part of the transaction. The Agencies have used consent orders to resolve competitive concerns about several of these mergers. Nonetheless, the Agencies have found some hospital mergers likely to have anticompetitive effects and had considerable early success in litigating hospital merger cases. From 1994 through 2000, however, when there were approximately 900 hospital mergers, the Agencies and state antitrust enforcers lost all seven cases they litigated. Some scholars have strongly criticized the courts' reasoning in these cases.

The Agencies analyse hospital mergers using the same

analytical framework they use for other mergers. The *1992 Horizontal Merger Guidelines (Merger Guidelines)* specify that "mergers should not be permitted to create or enhance market power or to facilitate its exercise." Market power "is the ability profitably to maintain prices above competitive levels for a significant period of time." A merger also may "lessen competition on dimensions other than price, such as product quality, service, or innovation."

To identify mergers that are likely to cause competitive problems, the *Merger Guidelines* provide for the examination of several issues, including:

- whether the merger, in light of market concentration and other factors that characterize the market, would be likely to have adverse competitive effects;
- whether entry would be timely, likely, and sufficient either to deter or to counteract the competitive effects of concern;
- whether there are efficiency gains from the merger that meet the Agencies' criteria for examination; and
- whether, but for the merger, either party to the transaction would be likely to fail, causing its assets to exit the market.

Merger analysis can begin with an assessment of direct evidence of likely anticompetitive effects. The Supreme Court has stated that "the finding of actual, sustained adverse effects on competition ... is legally sufficient to support a finding that the challenged restraint was unreasonable even in the absence of elaborate market analysis." A number of lower court decisions have followed this principle. Merger analysis also can begin with the identification of relevant product and geographic markets. A market is defined as a product(s) and a geographic area in which it is produced or sold, such that a hypothetical profit-maximising firm that was the only present and future producer or seller of those products in that area likely would impose at least a "small but significant and non-transitory" increase in price. This market definition test is sometimes referred to as the "hypothetical monopolist" paradigm. A relevant market is a group of products and a geographic area that is no bigger than necessary to satisfy this test. Analysis typically starts with a narrow area that is broadened until a price increase by the hypothetical firm would be profitable because consumers have insufficient substitution alternatives available to defeat it. Hospital merger analysis raises a number of significant issues, including how best to define the geographic and product markets, assess the prospects for entry and the likelihood and magnitude of efficiencies, and determine the relevance of a hospital's institutional status (for-profit or nonprofit). This chapter considers each of these issues, and discusses relevant case law, academic commentary and research, and testimony and written presentations from the Hearings. The role of group purchasing organisations (GPOs) for health care systems, including the extent to which GPOs act as agents of their buyer-members or as agents of the sellers that pay the GPOs' administrative fees. This section also discusses the antitrust issues GPOs may raise and the applicability of the *Health Care Statements* to those issues. A brief discussion of the antitrust implications of tiering and pay-for-performance.

II. Geographic Market Definition

The Agencies define hospital geographic markets using the process set forth in the *Merger Guidelines.* Panelists agreed that the *Merger Guidelines* provide an appropriate framework for defining and analysing hospital geographic markets. Although there is widespread agreement on the basic framework, two well-known health law scholars have written:

> [T]he law concerning hospital [geographic] market definition is in a shambles. Common sense suggests that health care, like politics, is local. In the words of Judge Richard Posner, "People want to be hospitalized near their families and homes, in hospitals in which their own - local - doctors have privileges." However, courts have stretched the geographic boundaries of

markets to strip merging hospitals of market power and thereby shield them from antitrust liability.

In this section, we discuss the controversies about how to define relevant geographic markets for hospitals. We discuss the use of the Elzinga-Hogarty test and critical loss analysis to define hospital geographic markets, including the views of proponents and critics. We then describe alternative analytical techniques and evidentiary sources that Hearing panelists and researchers proposed for defining hospital geographic markets. The final subsection summarizes the Agencies' conclusions and recommendations concerning geographic market definition issues. This subsection includes the conclusion that, to date, the Agencies' experience and research indicate that the Elzinga-Hogarty test is not valid or reliable in defining geographic markets in hospital merger cases. At the outset, we note that direct evidence of anticompetitive effects may make it unnecessary to define a relevant market. For example, consummated merger cases may present opportunities to assess competitive effects without using detailed market definitions.

A. Elzinga-Hogarty, Critical Loss, and the Alternatives

Since 1995, the Agencies have lost several hospital merger cases because the courts accepted the merging parties' use of patient flow data to perform either the Elzinga-Hogarty test or critical loss analysis to define the geographic market much more broadly than the plaintiff Agency. Commentators and panelists observed that these cases reflect judicial acceptance of implausibly large geographic markets, judicial approval of mergers that would not be permitted in any other industry, and the lessening of competition in the hospital services market. All panelists agreed that neither the parties nor the courts should use the Elzinga-Hogarty test as the sole basis for defining the geographic market. As one panelist stated: "if [Elzinga-Hogarty] is the only tool that is being used ... it blurs everyone's vision as to who really are the competitors and the alternatives that matter." Panelists and commentators identified numerous problems with the application of critical loss analysis, although panelists and commentators agreed that it can be a useful tool. Several panelists offered alternative analytical tools and other types of evidence to use in defining the geographic market for a hospital. Most panelists agreed that no one piece of information is sufficient to define a hospital's geographic market. In essence, panelists agreed the courts should apply the *Merger Guidelines'* hypothetical monopolist test in hospital merger cases, just as they do in merger cases involving other industries and products. The question is how to implement the hypothetical monopolist test, and what analytical frameworks and evidence should be used to do so.

1. Elzinga-Hogarty Test

The Elzinga-Hogarty test was designed to analyse commodity movements, not hospital mergers. It was proposed by two economists in an article critiquing the Agencies' geographic market definitions in two non-hospital merger cases. In one case, the government relied on LIFO ("little in from outside") data to argue that an entire state was the relevant geographic market for beer products. In the second case, the government relied on LOFI ("little out from inside") data to argue that the relevant geographic market for commercial banking was limited to a four-county area. Kenneth Elzinga and Thomas Hogarty argued that a proper geographic market analysis required the use of both LIFO and LOFI statistics, but observed that their analysis was not readily applicable to heterogenous goods or differentiated products. Hospitals generally provide heterogenous or differentiated goods and services.

Nonetheless, the "Elzinga-Hogarty test" has been used extensively in hospital merger cases. The movement of a patient who resides within the provisional geographic market to a facility outside of that area for hospital services is considered an importation of hospital services into that provisional geographic market, measured as LIFO. The movement of a patient who resides outside of the provisional geographic market to a facility inside the provisional geographic market for hospital services is considered an exporting of hospital services outside of the provisional geographical market, measured as LOFI. Thus, under the hospital application of the Elzinga-Hogarty test, evidence that few patients leave and few patients enter an area surrounding the merging hospitals is interpreted to support the conclusion that the area constitutes a relevant geographic market. Conversely, if the patient flow data show large numbers of patients coming into or going out of the area for inpatient hospital care, then the geographic market is hypothesized to be broader than originally thought, and must include hospitals further away from the merging hospitals. A geographic market definition is usually described as "strong" if less than 10 percent of discharged patients from the merging hospitals' area come into or out of the area. If more than 10 percent (but less than 25 percent) of patients migrate in or out of the hospitals' core geographic area for in-patient services, the market definition is considered "weak."

Panelists identified a number of weaknesses with the use of the Elzinga-Hogarty test to define a geographic market for hospital services. One panelist pointed out that the Elzinga-Hogarty test takes a leap in logic from a current level of patient migration to the conclusion that patients would respond to a small price increase by using hospitals outside of the merging hospitals' core geographic area - a leap not justified by either economic analysis or past experience. Patients decide whether or not to travel for health care services for a variety of reasons, including perceived and actual variations in quality, insurance coverage, out-of-pocket cost, sophistication of services, and family connections. Although patient flow data may show that patients go to hospitals beyond the core zip code area, this does not mean that their behaviour reflects price sensitivity, or that other consumers would travel if prices increased. Stated differently, patient flow data can show existing hospitalisation patterns, but offer no insight into what patients will do in response to a price increase by the merged hospital.

Another panelist described this phenomenon as the "silent majority fallacy."

> The E-H [Elzinga-Hogarty] approach draws a conclusion about the entire market from the behaviour of those consumers who express displeasure with their local sellers by traveling elsewhere. This is a valid logical leap when travelers and non-travelers have similar demands and related market experiences. However, if the two groups differ on dimensions other than location, then E-H gives rise to what we call the "silent majority fallacy." That is, if travelers and non-travelers display fundamentally different demand behaviour, either because they differ in their taste for travel or their need for local/nonlocal services, then there is no necessary relationship between the market experiences of these two groups post-merger. If travelers differ significantly from non-travelers, then the presence of a minority of travelers does not imply that local firms lack market power *vis-a-vis* the majority of consumers who are non-travelers.

The silent majority fallacy is a particular problem with hospital merger analysis, because the goods and services are not fungible commodities, but are "highly differentiated by location and other dimensions." Empirical evidence confirms that "the majority of patients are truly reluctant to travel and do not view distant hospitals as close substitutes for most services, even though a sizable percentage of their neighbors may travel for care. Those who do travel have distinct reasons for doing so and the fact that they travel would not inhibit merging local hospitals from increasing prices substantially."

One panelist also noted that in some circumstances, the Elzinga-Hogarty test cannot be satisfied. If the initial specification of the geographic market does not meet the required threshold for LIFO and LOFI, expanding the geographic market may not satisfy the required threshold either. The result is that the geographic market expands without limit. This problem alone casts serious doubt on the utility of the Elzinga-Hogarty methodology for hospitals. This same panelist suggested that the Elzinga-Hogarty test systematically leads to expansive geographic markets when zip codes are selected based on the absolute number of patients that come from a zip code. There is tremendous variability in the number of individuals that live in a particular zip code. A hospital may have a small share of total admissions from a particular zip code, even though it gets a significant number of patient admissions from that zip code - and the Elzinga-Hogarty test, as used in hospital mergers, will include such distant zip codes in the market. According to this panelist, "a zip code that has 20,000 people, that's 40 miles away, might get included if the hospital gets 50 patients from there, whereas ten zip codes that are closer that only have a thousand people each, might send 40 people each, they would get excluded." He suggested that such large and distant zip codes are particularly likely to be cities that have hospitals in them, which skews the results of the analysis from the outset.

2. Critical Loss Analysis

Critical loss analysis has the potential to provide a useful way to implement the hypothetical monopolist test, but it must be applied with great care. Problems with its application have led some commentators to question the value of critical loss analysis as an antitrust tool. Conventional critical loss analysis posits a particular price increase and asks what proportion of the hypothetical monopolist's sales would have to be lost to yield a net decrease in the hypothetical monopolist's profits. When critical loss analysis is used to delineate a relevant market, the first step is to calculate the percentage loss in sales that would make a given price increase unprofitable for a hypothetical monopolist over a candidate market. This calculation depends on the price increase posited and on the contribution margin (*i.e.*, price minus marginal cost, all divided by price) on the sales that would be lost. The second step is to estimate the likely actual loss in sales that would result from the hypothesized price increase, *e.g.*, what percentage of patients likely would stop patronizing the hospitals in the candidate market in response to the price increase. The estimated actual loss is then compared to the calculated critical loss. If the estimated actual loss exceeds the critical loss, it is inferred that the price increase would be unprofitable and the candidate market is too small to be a market. One panelist described misuses of the critical loss technique that practitioners should avoid. Notably, typical applications posit small *(e.g.,* five percent) price increases. Yet, the *Merger Guidelines'* methodology for delineation of relevant markets asks whether the profit-maximising price increase would be at least a small but significant amount *(e.g.,* five percent). Even though a monopolist may find a five percent price increase unprofitable, it may find a larger price increase profitable. This panelist presented an example based on the stylized facts of several hospital merger cases in which a five percent price increase would be unprofitable, but any price increase between 31 percent and 319 percent would be profitable, and the hypothetical monopolist would maximise its profits by increasing price 175 percent. Thus, the candidate market was a market under the *Merger Guidelines'* hypothetical monopolist test, even though a five percent price increase was unprofitable. This panelist discussed other problems that occur in some implementations of critical loss analysis. The standard formula presumes constant marginal cost and no avoidable fixed costs, but actual cost functions may differ significantly from this assumption. Also, the standard formula implicitly assumes proportionate increases in all prices, but the profit maximising strategy for hospitals may involve highly disproportionate price increases. This panelist also explained that critical loss calculations must focus on the margins for the patients that likely would be lost in the event of a price increase. Much of the potential for abuse in critical loss analysis involves the second step -estimation of the actual loss. Some practitioners have relied in inappropriate ways on consumer surveys or patient flow data to estimate the actual losses in sales that would result from a price increase. For example, some practitioners use patient flow data to identify zip codes that are "contestable."

These practitioners then argue that the share of patients in these zip codes that would stop patronizing certain hospitals in a candidate geographic market in response to a given price increase would be greater than the critical loss, and that the geographic area must therefore be expanded in order to constitute a relevant geographic market. Data on existing travel patterns for residents in a zip code, however, say nothing about why patients select specific hospitals or how a change in relative prices would affect patient migration. One cannot infer that just because some patients in a zip code currently choose more distant hospitals, others also would choose such hospitals if the prices of the merging hospitals increased.

Recent commentary, some of it published after the Hearings, has stressed a link between the first and second steps of critical loss analysis. As a simple matter of arithmetic, the higher the contribution margin, the smaller the critical loss will be for a given price increase. The higher the margin, the more it costs the hypothetical monopolist to lose a sale, and so the smaller the sales loss required to offset the profit gain from making the remaining sales at a higher price. Yet if firms are maximising profits before the merger, high margins indicate that those firms face low price elasticities of demand. Otherwise, these firms could earn greater total profits by *reducing* prices and expanding sales. Moreover, a hypothetical monopolist over any candidate market must face a lower elasticity of demand than the individual firms in that candidate market, so high margins must imply a very low demand elasticity for the candidate market. Hospitals' experts commonly argue that merging hospitals' margins are high, which implies that the critical losses are low. They argue that post-merger price increases would be unprofitable because of the high per-unit foregone profits on lost sales. In essence, they argue that where the critical loss is low, the actual loss will exceed the critical loss. On this basis, they argue that relevant geographic markets for hospital mergers are broad.

Yet, as discussed above, high margins also imply low demand elasticities. Low demand elasticities indicate that the merged firm's actual losses of sales would be low. Because the actual losses may be less than the critical losses when margins are high, the relevant geographic market may in fact be narrow. Other commentators also have described ways in which critical loss analysis has been carried out incorrectly, both for delineation of markets and for competitive effects analysis. One article cites four key problems in how courts have applied critical loss analysis in recent hospital mergers. First, courts have failed to consider whether a price increase greater than five percent would be profitable. Second, courts have failed to consider the fact that high margins often mean a firm faces inelastic demand and, therefore, actual losses would be low. Third, courts did not consider that, if prices increased, some consumers might be diverted to one of the merged firms. Finally, courts have assumed, contrary to economic theory, that firms in the area surrounding the merged firm would keep the same prices even though the merged firm raised its prices. Thus, critical loss analysis may be useful in defining geographic markets and for competitive effects analysis only if it is applied appropriately.

3. Alternative Analytical Techniques

One panelist proposed an alternative analytical framework built on the observation that hospitals compete in two stages. According to this panelist, the Agencies typically focus on first-stage competition, in which hospitals compete to be included in the networks of health plans. At this point, health plans are the buyers, and prices may be constrained if a health plan can credibly threaten to, or actually, exclude the merging hospitals from its provider network and divert patients to alternative hospitals. The focus for defining the geographic market for this first stage of competition is on hospital locations, not patient locations. Once a hospital is in the plan's network, or in some cases even if it is not, the hospitals then compete at the second stage - for the individual patient.

This panelist suggested that defendants typically focus on second-stage competition for patients and argue for broader geographic markets based on patient flow data. This level of competition differs significantly from the first stage. A two-stage analysis may result in different geographic markets and different competitive effects for each stage, because the two stages involve different customers, different means of competition, and different evidence. If anticompetitive effects are demonstrated at either stage, the merger should be enjoined, according to this panelist. Another panelist disagreed with the two-stage analysis, noting that it might be worth looking at "as a stylized construct," but that "the appropriate model in which to analyse the factors that drive the pricing decisions and the profitability decisions of the hospitals are such that one cannot separate out the two stages." She suggested that the distinction is even less relevant now, because most plans have inclusive provider networks. In these circumstances, network inclusion provides no assurance that patients will seek care at a particular hospital. Another panelist submitted a joint statement proposing a different analytical framework for analysing geographic markets in hospitals. The statement asserts that because potential patients select managed care organisations *(e.g.,* health insurers) prior to knowing what their medical needs will be, the subsequent *ex-ante* pricing makes the connection between patient flows and pricing power tenuous. For example, the statement suggests that "100% of patients place a high value on having access to a local hospital," but if they are part of the 20 percent of the group that develop a serious medical condition, these same patients may be willing to travel any distance to go to the best hospital for their condition. As an alternative, the statement proposes a formal demand analysis model that would require data on patient and hospital characteristics in addition to the patient origin and destination data traditionally used. Although this model is more complex than patient flow analysis, the statement contends it provides "a measure of market power that, unlike patient flows, is theoretically valid for differentiated goods markets and is directly related to the prices that hospitals are able to charge."

(B) Other Evidentiary Sources

Panelists suggested numerous additional sources of evidence that should be used to establish the geographic market for hospital services. The recommended sources include types of evidence typically assessed in non-hospital merger cases: strategic planning documents and testimony from the merging parties and their competitors, and documents and testimony from major purchasers of services from the merging parties - here, third-party payors. Panelists also suggested the use of evidence that casts direct light on the distances patients are willing to travel and the reasons they are willing to do so, and evidence that demonstrates the role, if any, physicians can play in defeating a hospital's post-merger, anticompetitive price increases. Each of these categories of evidence are considered below.

1. Hospital Strategic Planning Documents

The Agencies typically examine strategic planning documents from the merging parties and their competitors to assess relevant market and other key issues in merger analysis. Panelists suggested using strategic planning documents from the hospitals to help establish the proper geographic market. Such documents may specify the geographic regions in which a hospital is marketing its services and the hospitals it sees as its primary competition. In addition, a hospital's strategic planning documents frequently disclose the hospital management's assessment of the extent to which the proposed merger will increase the hospital's negotiating power and its ability to raise prices. Hospital strategic planning documents can illuminate hospital competition for both inclusion in payor networks and for individual patients.

2. Payor Testimony

For non-hospital mergers, the Agencies regularly obtain the views of the merging firms' major customers to assess issues such as relevant market definition and competitive effects. These market participants typically have the most price negotiation experience with the merging firms, as well as the most to lose from price increases (or quality or other degradations) if the proposed merger were to create market power. On the other hand, major customers also have much to gain from reduced prices if the proposed merger would likely create efficiencies that would be passed on to customers. Courts, however, have been skeptical about testimony from third-party payors in hospital merger cases, even though these payors routinely negotiate with hospitals about price and other aspects of hospital care. In *Tenet,* for example, the Eighth Circuit questioned the district court's reliance on payor testimony that they "would unhesitatingly accept a price increase rather than steer their subscribers to hospitals" outside of the core geographic area. The Eighth Circuit believed that, although the testimony might have been truthful, the payors "spoke to current competitor perceptions and consumer habits and failed to show where consumers could practicably go for inpatient hospital services." By contrast, panelists stated that payors can offer useful testimony on at least two distinct issues. Payors have considerable insight into hospital geographic markets, because they must factor such matters into their decision whether to contract with a hospital in the first instance. Payors must strive to include a sufficient number of hospitals in each geographic market, because if they fail to do so, the plan is less appealing to purchasers, including benefit managers that must make recommendations and decisions for employers and other group purchasers. Accordingly, payors can offer useful testimony on the extent to which particular hospitals engage in price and non-price competition with one another.

Second, panelists suggested that payor testimony also would be helpful in determining whether payors can steer patients to a lower-cost hospital if prices increase post-merger. Several panelists noted that payors used to create marketable plans with limited provider networks and thus could exclude a hospital if its prices were not acceptable to the plan. Today, many consumers demand choice and open provider networks. Therefore, payors frequently rely on mechanisms other than excluding hospitals to divert marginal consumers to lower-cost alternatives. For example, payors are currently experimenting with tiered networks that provide differing levels of coverage and co-payments based on the facility at which care is received. Testimony regarding the feasibility and performance of such strategies would be helpful in determining the alternatives available to payors in the event of post-merger price increases. Panelists expressed different views on whether and to what extent payors can "steer" patients and the types of evidence that can help answer this question. One panelist noted that if payors actually can steer patients to (or away) from particular institutions, the distances traveled to hospitals should have grown in parallel with the rise of managed care. In fact, the panelist noted, the distances patients travel to hospitals have not changed very much since the mid-1980s, and there is little distinction between the distances traveled for HMO versus non-HMO patients. Based on this evidence, the panelist maintained that courts should not assume that payors can effectively steer patients in response to price increases. Another panelist suggested that patient flow data may help show whether and, if so, how payors can steer patients. This panelist asserted that payors have had enough success in moving marginal consumers to lower-cost hospitals that, in most cases, they can discipline hospital price increases. She also concluded that in many cases, even if payors testify accurately that they must have the merging parties in their networks, that is not necessarily sufficient to give the hospitals unilateral power over price. Other panelists were more skeptical about these claims. One panelist stated that, although in theory payors have mechanisms they could use to divert patients to other hospitals, in practice these tactics are often costly and counter-productive to a health plan's marketability and profitability. This panelist argued that it is difficult (if not impossible) to target incentives to the insured consumers who are most likely to be affected. A pay or must consider the cost of providing a lower copayment to all patients, not just the marginal patients the pay or is trying to steer. Moreover, other hospitals may have higher prices than the merged hospitals, even assuming price increases as a result of the merger.

3. Patients' Willingness to Travel - How Far and Why?

Several panelists suggested that courts should give more weight to empirical studies of patients' willingness to travel to receive health care. Studies indicate that most patients prefer to be hospitalized close to their homes. Some patients appear willing to travel long distances for very serious or complicated procedures, but many patients prefer to receive such care in their local hospital, even if their local hospital has higher mortality rates and less experience with such procedures. Some patients are willing to receive care in a distant city because they work or have family in that city, or because of the hospital's religious affiliation. Several panelists noted that such migration patterns are unlikely to be price sensitive, yet the application of the Elzinga-Hogarty test and critical loss analysis would result in a large geographic market in such circumstances, if enough patients traveled for these non-price reasons.

4. Physicians' Willingness and Ability to Steer Patients to Less Expensive Alternatives

Several hearing participants suggested that payors may be able to provide financial incentives to physicians to steer patients to less expensive hospitals. Some of the proposals included requiring physicians to agree to a financial risk-sharing contract, threatening physicians with exclusion from a plan's network, imposing financial penalties on physicians who admit patients to the higher-priced hospitals, and providing bonuses to physicians who admit to lower-priced hospitals. Even though such incentives are theoretically possible, it does not follow that payors would find them useful or desirable. Indeed, such incentives could make a plan less marketable to employers and consumers who value open networks and unrestricted access to health care. Such incentives also could interfere with continuity of care, particularly if patients must use a different physician when they are diverted to a different hospital. These incentives also are unlikely to be effective if they require patients to travel long distances and physicians to travel those same distances to provide care.

(C) Summary

The definition of a relevant geographic market has proven to be one of the most daunting components of a hospital merger case. Nonetheless, some guiding principles are clear. The hypothetical monopolist test of the *Merger Guidelines* should be used to define geographic markets in hospital merger cases. The types of evidence used in *all* merger cases - such as strategic planning documents of the merging parties and customer testimony and documents -should also be used to delineate relevant geographic markets in hospital merger cases. The Agencies believe that courts have given insufficient weight to payor testimony and documents in particular. Empirical evidence is desirable on certain issues, such as the extent of patients' willingness to travel to distant hospitals in response to a small, but significant and non-transitory increase in price. Patient willingness to travel for non-price related reasons does not provide a sufficient basis to infer patient willingness to travel to distant hospitals in response to price increases.

The Agencies encourage further research to determine the circumstances in which patients will travel to distant hospitals in response to price increases. Empirical evidence also is desirable on the extent to which physicians can and will steer patients to lower-cost hospitals in response to price increases. To be persuasive, direct evidence should show that such steering by physicians is feasible, cost-effective, and likely. The Agencies also encourage additional research to validate or refute the alternative analytical techniques discussed *supra.* To date, and for the reasons discussed *supra,* the Agencies' experience and research indicate that the Elzinga-Hogarty test is not valid or reliable in defining geographic markets in hospital merger cases. In addition, if critical loss analysis is used, it must be used with great care to avoid the problems of application discussed in this section. The use of the Elzinga-Hogarty test and the misapplication of critical loss analysis has led some courts to find hospital geographic markets that are improbably large.

III. Product Market Definition

The *Merger Guidelines* provide the framework for defining the relevant product market for hospital services. The product market has typically been defined as a broad group of medical and surgical diagnostic and treatment services for acute medical conditions where the patient must remain in a health care facility for at least 24 hours for recovery or observation. Over the past twenty years, many hospital merger cases have considered and rejected outpatient services as part of the relevant product market for hospitals. For example, in *In re Hospital Corp. of America,* 106 F.T.C. 361 (1985), the Commission noted that, although outpatient care for certain services might be a separate relevant market or markets, the evidence demonstrated "that the core and vast majority of an acute care hospital's business is acute inpatient care" and non-hospital outpatient providers could not defeat post-merger anticompetitive behaviour affecting hospital inpatients.

The Seventh Circuit agreed, observing that "although hospitals increasingly are providing services on an out-patient basis ... most hospital services cannot be provided by nonhospital providers; as to these, hospitals have no competition from other providers of medical services." Similarly, in *American*

Medical International, 104F.T.C. 1 (1984), the Commission excluded outpatient services from the product market. The Eleventh Circuit also accepted inpatient acute-care services as the relevant product market in *University Health.* Only one court has included outpatient providers within the product market for inpatient services.

Panelists agreed that providers of outpatient services, such as physicians' offices, urgent care centers, and ambulatory surgery centers, should generally not be included in the product market definition for hospital services. Panelists indicated that from the perspective of payors and patients, inpatient services are complementary and bundled. Even if hospital prices are increased, patients and payors cannot separate nursing care, diagnostic tests, and room and board from the other treatments provided as part of a hospital stay and outsource them. Similarly, demand-side substitution is improbable; a cancer or heart attack patient is not going to substitute obstetrical care if prices for cancer care or heart attacks increase. Because outpatient treatment is generally not a substitute for inpatient care, there was agreement among the panelists that outpatient providers are (and were) correctly excluded from the product market. In the future it is likely that the Agencies will have to determine whether certain specialty hospitals should be included in an inpatient product market for particular proposed hospital mergers. Historically, the type of specialty hospital (children's, psychiatric, VA, military, and rehabilitation) justified its exclusion from the product market. In recent years, specialty hospitals focusing on cardiac or orthopedic care have emerged in numerous locations. General acute-care hospitals view these specialty hospitals as competition in the provision of such services and have responded in a variety of ways.

Several panelists discussed an approach for defining an inpatient hospital product market more narrowly. Instead of treating acute inpatient treatment as an aggregated group, panelists suggested the possibility of grouping diagnosis related groups (DRGs) together, based upon the types of diseases and medical conditions treated by particular types of physicians. In one study, this approach resulted in 48 service categories. Patient flow data can be separately analysed for each category. Panelists recognized, however, that payors generally do not disaggregate services this finely. Although the Agencies currently doubt the advisability and practicability of conducting separate product market analyses for many discrete markets - particularly when payors do not define the product they are purchasing in this fashion - the Agencies will continue to examine whether smaller product markets exist in addition to the traditional product market definition. For example, if more specialized medical procedures raise more competitive concerns than primary care services, there may be some circumstances in which the product market should be defined narrowly to include only a specific service or limited number of services. Similarly, it is possible that expertise in one or more specific specialities may make a hospital a "must have" hospital for a payor's network, which could justify a separate product market analysis.

IV. Entry

The *Merger Guidelines* provide that entry should be considered if it is likely to occur within two years and to be sufficient to deter or counteract anticompetitive effects of a proposed hospital merger. Entry into the inpatient general acute care hospital services market by constructing a new hospital or adding additional beds to an existing facility is likely to exceed this time-frame. If the state requires that a Certificate of Need (CON) be granted before building a new hospital or increasing bed capacity, the approval of the CON can take anywhere from 18 months to several years. Compliance with other regulations will require additional time. Thus, the likelihood of timely and sufficient entry into the inpatient general acute care hospital services market is remote.

V. Efficiencies

The *Merger Guidelines* make clear that efficiencies should

be evaluated before determining whether a proposed merger is likely to be pro- or anti-competitive. Under the *Merger Guidelines,* the Agencies will not challenge a merger if cognizable efficiencies are of a character and magnitude such that the merger is not likely to be anticompetitive in any relevant market. Efficiencies are cognizable when they are (1) merger-specific, (2) have been verified, and (3) do not arise from anticompetitive reductions in output or service.

Hospitals often claim that their merger will produce significant efficiencies, and some courts have given significant weight to these arguments. Claimed efficiencies have included avoidance of capital expenditures, reductions in management and operational support jobs, consolidation of specific services to one location *(e.g.,* all cardiac care at Hospital A and all cancer treatments at Hospital B), and reducing operational costs, such as purchasing and accounting. Some hospitals claim that after the merger they will be able to provide better and more complex services to their patients. For example, in *Tenet* the merging hospitals claimed they would realise significant efficiencies, including: eliminating unused beds, bringing open heart surgery to Poplar Bluff, decreasing operating costs, consolidating services, reducing staff levels, and avoiding capital expenditures. The district court rejected the hospitals' efficiency claims. The Eighth Circuit found that, although the district court may have properly rejected the hospitals' efficiencies, it should have nonetheless considered the claim that the merged entity would provide better care to its patients. The appellate court stated that "[t]he reality of the situation in our changing healthcare environment may be that Poplar Bluff cannot support two high-quality hospitals;" and admonished the district court for placing "an inordinate emphasis on price competition."

Some panelists were skeptical about efficiency claims. Several panelists pointed out that promised efficiencies may not materialize. One panelist noted that efficiency studies are often conducted to support the HSR filing that the merging parties must make with the Agencies; this provides incentives for the parties to estimate unrealistically high savings. Another noted that mergers can be great failures if hospitals do not have specific plans or are not willing to make tough decisions at the outset, such as closing facilities and consolidating hospital-based physician groups. Institutional constraints can make it difficult for merged hospitals to combine and coordinate clinical operations. For example, in *Butterworth,* the district court accepted the merging hospitals' claims that the proposed merger would result in efficiencies in excess of $100 million in the form of capital expenditure avoidance and operating efficiencies. One panelist reported, however, that Blodgett/Butterworth never closed Blodgett and consolidated services, at least in part because physician groups did not want the facility closed. Another panelist stated that, six years after the merger, Blodgett/Butterworth had realised less than half of the $100 million of claimed efficiencies.

Scholars have conducted numerous studies on the effect of hospital mergers on hospital costs. The results are mixed: some studies have found that merged hospitals enjoy lower costs (or lower rates of cost increase) than nonmerging hospitals; others have found no differences in cost experience between merging hospitals and otherwise similar nonmerging facilities. One recent study found that the degree of cost savings that merging hospitals realise varies significantly depending on the extent of consolidation. According to this study, hospitals operating under a single license post-merger generate "significant, robust, and persistent" savings. In contrast, those hospitals that conduct business under separate licences post-merger do not generate cost reductions. The authors attribute this difference to the ability of more fully merged hospitals to undertake substantial changes in they way they operate (including consolidation of services) that are not available to hospitals operating under separate licenses. Even if a hospital merger is likely to create cognizable efficiencies, those cognizable efficiencies likely will not be sufficient to reverse a hospital merger's potential to harm consumers in the relevant market by preventing price increases in that market.

As discussed, *supra,* most studies of the relationship between competition and hospital prices generally find that increased hospital concentration is associated with increased prices. Some panelists and commentators believe an important motivation for the creation of multi-hospital systems has been to gain market power to secure higher reimbursement from payors. Indeed, one academic health economist reported that "I have asked many providers why they wanted to merge. Although publicly they all invoked the synergies mantra, virtually everyone stated privately that the main reason for merging was to avoid competition and/or obtain market power."

In several merger cases, hospitals have signed "community commitments" or agreements with State Attorneys General, promising not to raise prices for a specified period or to pass onto consumers a specified amount of money from the claimed efficiencies. Some State Attorneys General have signed these agreements in an attempt to translate merger-induced cost savings into price reductions to consumers. For example, in *Butterworth / Blodgett,* the merging hospitals agreed: (1) to freeze list prices for three years, (2) to freeze prices for managed care plans at pre-merger levels, (3) to limit profit margins by targeting a five-year rolling average for the merged entity that would not exceed the average of Moody's and Standard & Poor's upper quartile profit margin for other national health care providers, (4) to serve the medically needy, and (5) to ensure that the board of the merged entity would continue to reflect the interests of western Michigan. Similarly, the merging hospitals in *Long Island Jewish Medical Center* entered into an agreement with the Attorney General of the State of New York to "pass on to the community cost savings that will be achieved . . . [to] equal 100 million dollars during the five-year period commencing January 1, 1998." The agreement further provided that up to 50 million dollars of the cost savings could be used "to fulfill its mission to provide high quality health care to economically disadvantaged and elderly members of the community." Community commitments are temporary and may not represent a binding constraint even during the period they are in effect. Furthermore, such commitments do not solve the underlying competitive problem when a hospital merger has changed market circumstances in ways that increase the likelihood that market power will be exercised. Community commitments represent a distinctly regulatory approach to what is, at bottom, a problem of competition - and that problem will remain after the commitment has expired. The Agencies do not accept community commitments as a resolution to likely anticompetitive effects from a hospital (or any other) merger. The Agencies believe community commitments are an ineffective short-term regulatory approach to what is ultimately a problem of competition. Nevertheless, the Agencies realise that in some circumstances, State Attorneys General may agree to community commitments in light of the resource and other constraints they face.

VI. Nonprofit Status of Hospitals

The significance of institutional form (nonprofit v. for-profit) has been an issue in several hospital merger cases. In three early cases, the Seventh and Eleventh Circuit Courts of Appeals rejected the claim that institutional form should figure in a merger analysis. Thus, in *HCA,* the Seventh Circuit noted that although "different ownership structures might reduce the likelihood of collusion, ... this possibility is conjectural," and that "adoption of the nonprofit form does not change human nature." Similarly, in *University Health,* the Eleventh Circuit observed that "the Supreme Court has rejected the notion that nonprofit corporations act under such a different set of incentives than for-profit corporations that they are entitled to an implicit exemption from the antitrust laws." Finally, in *Rockford,* the Seventh Circuit repeated and elaborated its position that institutional form was irrelevant to a merger analysis:

> We are aware of no evidence - and the [appellees] present none, only argument - that nonprofit suppliers of goods or services are more likely to compete vigorously than profit-making suppliers .... If the managers of nonprofit enterprises are less likely to strain after that last penny of profit, they may be less prone to engage in profit-maximising collusion but by the same token less prone to engage in profit-maximising competition.

The relevant question for antitrust analysis is not whether nonprofit hospitals behave in a manner indistinguishable from for-profit institutions, but rather whether they would exploit merger-created market power in ways harmful to consumers. Recently, some courts have asserted that institutional form should matter - and suggested that nonprofit hospitals, even if they acquire market power, will not harm competition or consumers. For example, in *Butterworth,* the district court relied on the nonprofit status of the merging hospitals as a reason why the merger would not have anticompetitive effects, and the Sixth Circuit emphasized this fact in its opinion affirming the district court.

Similarly, in *Long Island Jewish Medical Center,* the court believed that the merging hospitals were nonprofit organisations that "have a genuine commitment to help their communities," and "community service, not profit maximisation, is the hospitals' mission." The practical significance of a hospital's institutional form has been studied extensively. One panelist (who was an expert for the defendant in the *Butterworth / Blodgett* case) stated that economic incentives made it likely that a typical nonprofit hospital's pricing behaviour would differ systematically from that of a typical for-profit hospital. This panelist argued that a number of studies, including work he had performed, indicated that nonprofits that attain market power behave differently from for-profits when it comes to pricing. This panelist qualified this observation, noting that the observed price effects in these studies are averages and do not predict whether or not a particular nonprofit hospital merger will have an effect on price and do not preclude the possibility of price discrimination against certain customers. Moreover, this panelist acknowledged that the empirical evidence of a price effect is mixed.

By contrast, several panelists maintained that the best available empirical evidence indicated no significant differences between the pricing behaviour of for-profit and nonprofit hospitals. For example, one panelist stated that "the preponderance of the empirical evidence indicates that nonprofit hospitals use their market power in roughly the same fashion as for-profit hospitals." Another panelist similarly reported that the "literature suggests that, on average, nonprofit hospitals do use market power to obtain higher prices." Recent empirical studies of pricing behaviour paint a fairly consistent picture. One study found that there was no significant difference in how for-profit and nonprofit hospitals exerted market power; for-profit hospitals generally had higher prices in 1986, but nonprofits increased their prices faster from 1986 to 1994. A case study of a nonprofit hospital merger in Santa Cruz, California, found significant evidence of post-merger price increases. Another study noted that "the most interesting result for antitrust policy is the finding that nonprofit hospital mergers lead to higher prices, not lower ones, and that the price increases resulting from a nonprofit merger are getting larger over time."

Merger simulation studies have produced a similar picture. One study found nonprofit status did not lead to lower prices in urban markets, but did result in modestly lower prices in rural markets. Other studies found no differences in pricing behaviour resulting from institutional status. One panelist asserted that even if there are no pricing differences between for-profit and nonprofit hospitals, there can be other differences. Nonprofit hospitals may have different long-term missions and have a different level of public accountability because of their long-term community obligations. There is some empirical evidence that institutional status affects the mix of services provided by a hospital.

This panelist also suggested that board members of a for-profit hospital had fiduciary duties to a different group of individuals than would be the case if the hospital was nonprofit.Another panelist responded that "ownership variations are distinctions without a significant difference [and that all hospitals, irrespective of ownership] have the same mission: to provide the highest quality, appropriate medical care possible to the patients they serve, irrespective of the patient's ability to pay for such care." Government statistics indicate that on average, uncompensated care accounts for a similar percentage of total costs at for-profit and nonprofit hospitals. Although institutional status has loomed large in debates and legal disputes, the best available evidence indicates that nonprofits exploit market power when given the opportunity to do so. Accordingly, the profit/nonprofit status of the merging hospitals should not be considered a factor in predicting whether a hospital merger is likely to be anticompetitive.

VII. Group Purchasing Organisations

A group purchasing organisation (GPO) negotiates contracts with vendors of medical supplies on behalf of its members. GPO members include hospitals, nursing homes, home health agencies, and other health care systems. Some Hearing participants and industry commentators assert that GPOs, acting as their members' buying cooperatives, can be tremendous engines of efficiency, allowing medical buyers to pool their purchasing power to lower health care costs.

Nonetheless, others assert that certain GPO contracting practices may raise competitive concerns related to tying, bundling, and exclusive dealing. The Senate Judiciary Committee, through efforts by Chairman Mike DeWine and Ranking Member Herb Kohl of the Antitrust, Competition Policy and Consumer Rights Subcommittee, and the U.S.

General Accounting Office have examined this issue in depth, and the issue was an important topic in the Hearings and the Commission's Health Care Workshop.

In the sections that follow, we explain what a GPO is, describe its role as a purchasing intermediary, and provide an overview of the GPO industry structure. This section then discusses the various organisational structures GPOs may adopt, the potential incentives created by each, and the various contracting practices used by either GPOs or their suppliers and their potential impact on competition.

Finally, this section addresses concerns expressed during the Hearings and elsewhere that *Health Care Statement* 7, which governs GPOs, impedes the Agencies' ability to challenge GPO practices when, and if, they are anticompetitive. For the reasons discussed below, the Agencies believe these concerns are misplaced, and it is not necessary to revise *Health Care Statement* 7. This statement does not provide a safety zone for the specific types of conduct that some commentators have criticized, including tying, bundling, or exclusive dealing. In such situations, the Agencies would analyse the conduct on a case-by-case basis to determine whether it may violate the antitrust laws.

(A) What is a GPO?

GPOs are entities that aggregate health care providers' purchasing volume and contracting functions to negotiate discounts with manufacturers, distributors, and other vendors of medical products and services. According to the Health Industry Group Purchasing Association (HIGPA), 96 percent of all acute care hospitals in the United States use the services of a GPO, and on average, hospitals use at least two GPOs. More than 70 percent of hospital purchases are made through a contract negotiated by a GPO. GPOs negotiate contracts with manufacturers of products that fall into two general categories - commodities and medical devices. Cotton balls, bandages, and linens are examples of commodities for which hospital clinical staffs generally do not have strong preferences about the manufacturer. High technology medical devices such as pacemakers and stents are examples of medical devices for which hospital clinicians may have a preference as to the manufacturer.

GPOs are not wholesalers or distributors, and they do not take possession of, or title to, the products for which they negotiate contracts. Vendors of medical supplies and services generally submit bids to a GPO in response to a "Request For Proposal." One panelist stated that GPOs "simply negotiate a contract with a supplier that all members of the GPO can access. This guarantees the GPO member that it will receive a price no worse than the pre-negotiated price on the GPO contract." Hospitals and other health care providers then purchase products and services directly from the vendor pursuant to the prices and contract terms specified in the GPO's contract with that vendor. Others note that in many cases, the GPO's contract does not bind the health care providers and they are free to negotiate separately with the vendor. According to one commentator, "GPO members have substantial freedom to purchase alternative products and do so in significant volumes, particularly where the products in question are differentiated."

(B) GPO Industry Overview

The Hospital Bureau of New York, established in 1910, is the first known hospital GPO. According to HIGPA, "[f]rom 1974 to 1999, the number of GPOs grew from forty to 633 . . . [and] it is estimated that approximately 200 GPOs contract directly with suppliers, and that twenty-six of these operate on a national level." One commentator asserted that "when markets in this industry are properly defined, no GPO has a market share as high as 20%. Further, there are many GPOs, and hospitals can and do join multiple GPOs or switch memberships." In contrast, the GAO's pilot study focused on seven national GPOs, each with purchasing volume of more than $1 billion. The GAO stated that the seven GPOs collectively accounted for purchases totaling approximately $43 billion, or "more than 85% of all hospital purchases nationwide made through GPO contracts." Moreover, according to the GAO, the two largest GPOs in its study accounted for approximately 66 percent of total GPO purchasing. One panelist explained that the numbers may differ depending on the study, the years measured, and whether percentages are based on all hospital purchases or only on hospital purchases made through a GPO. For example, this panelist noted that the largest GPO accounts for 15 percent of total purchases by hospitals, but 30 percent of purchases made by hospitals through a GPO. Similarly, the second largest GPO's market share goes from 12 percent of all purchases to 25 percent of purchases made through a GPO.

(C) Structure and Incentives

The GAO report explained that "GPOs differ in their corporate structures and their relationships with member hospitals." Member hospitals own some GPOs; in other cases, shareholders that are independent of the member hospitals own the GPO. In some instances, suppliers finance GPOs by paying administrative fees that often are calculated as a percentage of each member's purchases of each supplier's products. These fees are designed to "cover [a] GPO's operating expenses and serve[] as its main source of revenue." GPOs may distribute surplus fees to their member hospitals as well. GPOs may be for-profit or nonprofit organisations.

Because of these differing structures, some panelists and commentators question the extent to which GPOs act as the agents of their buyer-members, or as the agents of the sellers that pay the GPOs' administrative fees. Because suppliers pay GPO fees, some worry that GPOs may operate to increase suppliers' revenues - and, correspondingly, GPO fees - rather than to minimize members' purchasing costs. Some panelists stated that when GPO members play important decision-making roles in the GPO, the GPO may be more likely to act as the agent of its buyer members. As one commentator put it, "[m]any GPOs are owned by their members, who sit on their boards, and are operated as cooperatives. These boards have no interest in procuring overpriced or substandard products [on] behalf of their own institutions." Similarly, one CEO stated that in his GPO the buyers

> make all of the [GPO] contracting decisions ... [award] all of the contract[s] ... decide which suppliers get the contracts, what their compliance requirements are going to be, ... [and] the type of contract that's going to be awarded, whether it's a sole source contract, a dual source contract, or a multi-source contract... [and that each health care system] has a seat on [the] Board of Directors ... see[s] financial statements every month, ... help[s] us set the budget... [and has] a seat on every single contracting body.

Another panelist stated that hospitals in such GPOs have "multiple opportunities through surveys, through advisory boards, advisory groups ... to have input into the suppliers that are selected for contract in [their] group purchasing organisation."

Other panelists asserted, however, that some GPOs act as the agents of the suppliers. One panelist asserted that the majority of GPOs "are financed and thereby controlled by large medical product companies rather than by the hospitals they are supposedly the agents for .... Fees and other incentives running from large medical manufacturers to GPOs allow such manufacturers to inappropriately influence the buying policies of the GPOs, because the compensation of most GPO management is almost always based on this fee income rather than on the real savings to hospital members." As a result, another contended, GPOs "are selling protected market share to dominant suppliers in exchange for fees." Such seller payments "may reflect side-payments being made in exchange for the GPOs conferring a de facto exclusivity that enhances the market power of the incumbent device maker."

(D) Contracting Practices

At the Hearings, panelists focused a significant portion of the discussion on whether certain GPO contracting practices - principally alleged tying, bundling, or exclusive dealing practices - injure competition. Such contracting practices include allegations that GPOs negotiate sole-source contracts with certain privileged manufacturers; require hospitals to purchase given volumes of certain supplies; bundle contracts that offer price discounts to purchasers of particular product groups; and enter contracts with manufacturers that last five years or more. GPOs' critics stated that some suppliers, in league with GPOs with sufficiently large market share, can insist upon a variety of anticompetitive GPO contracting practices to exclude rival suppliers from serving the buyers. They argue that such practices can discourage competitors from entering to bring down prices, and can discourage the research and development efforts necessary to produce innovative health care products that may improve on the incumbent's product. Some charge, for example, that "if a large GPO negotiates a sole-source contract with a manufacturer, the contract could cause an efficient, competing manufacturer to lose business and exit from the market and could discourage other manufacturers from entering the market."

Similarly, GPOs' critics challenge hospital "commitments" to purchase a given volume to obtain a better price. According to one panelist, under such a commitment, a hospital that buys an unauthorized product not only loses its better price on the complying product, but also must repay savings earned from having enjoyed that better price for years. Critics also challenge contracts that offer bundled price discounts to purchasers of particular product groups, and contracts of five years or more that "can direct business to manufacturers for an extended period."

The economic literature on tying, bundling, and exclusive dealing practices indicates that they can be efficient, although under certain circumstances they may be harmful to competition. Scholarly legal commentary in recent years also has called into question the anticompetitive explanations for these practices and has focused on efficiencies and the potential welfare-enhancing aspects of these business arrangements. Thus, courts typically engage in a fact-intensive inquiry to evaluate the competitive effects of such tying, bundling, and exclusive dealing claims.

Courts reviewing tying claims generally require that "(1) two separate products or services are involved, (2) the sale or agreement to sell one is conditioned on the purchase of the other, (3) the seller has sufficient economic power in the market for the tying product to enable it to restrain trade in the market for the tied product, and (4) a not insubstantial amount of interstate commerce in the tied product is affected." Courts reviewing the competitive consequences of exclusive dealing contracts typically analyse factors such as:

> the degree of exclusion flowing from the restraint, its duration and terminability, the percentage of the market foreclosed and other indicia of the likely effect on competitors' ability to operate, the availability of alternative access routes to supplies or customers, rivals' ability to employ countermeasures to defeat the attempted exclusion, and, ultimately, the likely impact of raising rivals' costs on competition in a relevant market, including consideration of any procompetitive justifications.

As a threshold matter, some panelists and commentators questioned whether allegations of exclusive dealing, tying, and bundling are true. For example, one panelist stated that "very few GPO contracts today are, in fact, exclusive," and unlike true exclusive dealing contracts, sole source contracts allow hospitals the freedom to buy from others. Another commentator noted that GPO loyalty rebate programs allow buyers to purchase from rivals offering lower prices. Other panelists noted that many long-term contracts are qualified in that "almost all GPO contracts can be terminated on 60- to 90-days notice."

Some panelists argued that, even if the GPOs were doing what their critics alleged, these contracting practices can actually increase, not decrease, consumer welfare. For example, one source reported that GPOs use the challenged contracting practices "as incentives for manufacturers to provide deeper discounts and for hospital members to concentrate purchasing volume to obtain better prices." Some researchers and industry representatives claim that providers who make purchases pursuant to GPO contracts generally save 10 to 15 percent of the price they would otherwise pay. Also, GPO contracts that bundle products can be "simply ways of making products more attractive, effectively cutting price, or reducing costs by disposing of excess inventory."

One panelist asserted that programs that allow suppliers to "reward [buyers'] higher levels of compliance" can be procompetitive "because they're offering increased dividends in exchange for volume," and because they standardize the buyers' products, which "leads to lower inventory costs [and] the ability to standardize patient care, leading to better quality, better staff education and improved safety." This same panelist explained that long-term contracts are sometimes necessary in light of the costs of "large clinical evaluations." He explained the process involved for clinically evaluating a particular product:

> The evaluation took 18 months. Our direct costs were over $150,000 .... We looked at product utilisation in over 8,500 surgical cases in 60 of our facilities with over 2,100 surgeons participating. At the end of that evaluation process, our owners said this was too much work to award just a three-year contract... [and] they decided to award a five-year contract.

He further stated that "strong" GPO programs are needed to counter the growing market power of suppliers that have consolidated in recent years. Finally, he also questioned whether the challenged practices could really be injuring the upstream supplier market, citing evidence that the medical device market is flourishing. Others, however, question GPOs' claimed efficiencies. For example, after a pilot study, the General Accounting Office reported that "GPOs' prices were not always lower and were often higher than prices paid by hospitals negotiating with vendors directly."

According to the GPO industry, GPOs provide additional benefits to their members, including reduced overhead costs for purchasing departments. In addition, GPOs claim to provide "assistance with product-comparison analysis and standardisation of products." Through GPOs, members may be able to reduce their supply costs via group purchasing, rebates, and surplus dividend payments.

As one panelist stated, GPOs can not only "eliminate wasteful administrative duplication[,]. they increase competition between rival GPOs, manufacturers and their member hospitals, all of which can translate into lower prices and higher quality for consumers." Moreover, "GPOs assist members in product selection, an activity that would otherwise use up large amounts of member staff time." One estimate suggested that hospitals would spend on average $155,000 per hospital to duplicate the administrative and other functions GPOs provide. The structure and incentives of individual GPOs may play an important role in determining the level of efficiencies they obtain. For example, GPOs acting on their members' behalf may strive to achieve efficiencies for the members. Thus, some noted that when the challenged contracting practices are arranged not by one rival manufacturer seeking to foreclose others, but by "a buyer or its agent" - *i.e.,* the buyers or their GPO - "in order to get lower prices from the manufacture[r]," the practices are likely to be pro-competitive.

One panelist suggested this circumstance distinguishes the challenged practices from typical tying and bundling cases. Indeed, another panelist believed that a GPO's refusal to carry a given manufacturer's product likely reflects buyers' skepticism about the manufacturer's claims about its product, not any competitive injury. By contrast, some commentators suggest that if suppliers control a GPO, the organisation may lack the incentive to promote efficiencies for its members. Some panelists suggested that such GPOs may have an incentive to collude with suppliers aiming to injure rival suppliers in a bid to acquire market power over the market for providing goods and services to the buyers. Under this theory, the GPOs agree to raise barriers against rival suppliers through contract terms imposing tying, bundling, or exclusive dealing arrangements on the buyers. These terms seek to "exclude rival manufacturers from competing for hospital sales even when the rival products are better or cheaper." Although suppliers do not need GPO support to attempt to exclude their rivals from the downstream market, one panelist suggested that the GPOs can streamline the efforts to exclude.

GPO members may also find it difficult to pursue other means of procuring goods for a variety of reasons. For example, member hospitals may be contractually bound to purchase certain supplies through a given GPO; the efficiencies that GPOs afford may outweigh their anticompetitive costs; member hospitals may enjoy "side-payments or special discounts" that give them private incentives to stay; a race-to-the-bottom effect may persuade a hospital to maintain its special GPO discount so that it does not suffer *vis-a-vis* its rivals; or agency problems that reward hospital administrators for winning short-term price cuts regardless of long-term harms may prevent hospitals from taking action against these anticompetitive practices.

Others counter that GPOs are unlikely to collude with suppliers in this way for long, because buyers unhappy with the anticompetitive results can always leave the GPO for other means of purchasing supplies. One panelist noted that GPOs must compete for hospitals' business and that hospitals "are free to select GPOs that best represent their interests."

E. Statement 7 Does Not Protect Anticompetitive Contracting Practices

Health Care Statement *7 addresses the formation of a GPO. Some have proposed altering* Statement 7, *citing to concerns about alleged anticompetitive contracting practices. The Agencies, however, do not believe that it is appropriate or wise to amend* Statement 7, *because the statement and its safety zone thresholds do not prevent and should not be appropriately read as preventing antitrust challenges to any of the alleged anticompetitive contracting practices about which panelists and others have raised concerns.*

> **Health Care Statement**
>
> This statement provides in part: "The Agencies will not challenge, absent extraordinary circumstances, any joint purchasing arrangement among health care providers where two conditions are present: (1) the purchases account for less than 35 percent of the total sales of the purchased product or service in the relevant market; and (2) the cost of the products and services purchased jointly accounts for less than 20 percent of the total revenues from all products or services sold by each competing participant in the joint purchasing arrangement."

Statement 7 and its safety zone thresholds aim to address monopsony and oligopoly concerns with the formation of a GPO. This statement reflects concerns that a particular GPO could (1) create monopsony power, injuring competition in the supplier market or (2) facilitate collusion in the sale of hospital products or services, injuring competition in the downstream market.

Statement 7 *does not address all potential issues that GPOs may raise. For example, it is silent on alleged exclusive dealing, tying, and bundling concerns that many panelists discussed in the Hearings. It is also silent on other potential competitive concerns, such as price-fixing, market allocation, mergers, etc. No statement is likely to cover every issue that could arise. The Agencies believe amending the statement to address some, but not all potential issues, is likely to be counterproductive. For example, some might argue that because certain issues were discussed,* Statement 7 *implicitly endorses as legal whatever conduct is not specifically addressed. If a supplier coordinates with the buyers, or with GPOs that have turned on their buyers, to exclude rival suppliers,* Statement 7 *would not protect such conduct from antitrust challenge.* In sum, *Statement* 7 governs Agency actions examining monopsony and oligopoly issues in connection with a GPO's formation. It does not preclude Agency action challenging anticompetitive conduct - such as anticompetitive contracting practices - that happens to occur in connection with GPOs. The Agencies will examine, on a case-by-case basis, the facts of any alleged anticompetitive contracting practices to determine whether the practice violates the antitrust laws.

VIII. Tiering and Pay-for-Performance

Commentators and panelists noted that some providers have resisted tiering and pay-for-performance programs, and refused to provide information regarding the quality of care they provide. When providers collectively refuse to enter into such arrangements or provide information to purchasers, the Agencies will carefully examine such conduct. As appropriate, the Agencies will bring cases against providers who collusively refuse to enter into such arrangements or provide such information. The Agencies also will challenge unilateral conduct or bundled contracting practices, where appropriate.

INDUSTRY SNAPSHOT AND COMPETITION LAW: PHYSICIANS

I. Overview

Competition has spurred significant changes in the market for physician services in the past several decades. How many physicians have sought to use innovative joint ventures to provide consumers with higher quality care at lower prices, while others have sought to stifle competition through conduct such as price-fixing and restrictions on allied health professionals. Reflecting consumer concerns about the quality, availability, and price of physician services, we highlight the benefits to consumers of competitive markets and vigorous antitrust enforcement. This study considers two types of provider network joint ventures - independent practice associations (IPAs) and physician-hospital organizations (PHOs) - that are part of the rapidly changing marketplace for physician services. We then discuss physician payment arrangements, the messenger model, and physician collective bargaining. Next, the chapter evaluates the competitive impact of restricting physicians' and allied health professionals' market entry. Finally, we examine the application of antitrust law to certain aspects of the marketplace for physician services, including private antitrust litigation about credentialing, the Agencies' analysis to assess the financial and clinical integration of joint ventures, and the ability of physicians to share and use information relating to quality improvements. Representatives from physician groups and organizations, attorneys, economists, and scholars testified on these matters over seven days of Hearings. Physician topic panels included Health Care Services: Provider Integration (September 9, 2002); Physician Hospital Organizations (May 8); Quality and Consumer Information: Physicians (May 30); Quality and Consumer Protection: Market Entry (June 10); Prospective Guidance (June 26); Physician Product and Geographic Market Definition (September 24); Physician Information Sharing (September 24); Physician IP As: Patterns and Benefits of Integration (September 25); Physician IP As: Messenger Model (September 25); and Physician Unionization (September 26).

II. Introduction

Spending on physician and clinical services accounts for approximately 22% of the $1.6 trillion spent annually on health care services. Total spending on physician services increased at an average annual rate of 12 percent from 1970-1993. Spending on physician services is projected to increase approximately seven percent per year for the next decade. Nevertheless, the percentage of national health spending devoted to physician services is likely to decline given "[t]he continued shift of care to other professional services, negative updates to the Medicare physician payment rates, and raster growth in other sectors such as prescription drugs." Although physician services account for only 22 percent of total health care spending, the treatment decisions of physicians profoundly affect both the cost and quality of the other health care services that consumers receive. The cost and geographic distribution of physician services affect the accessibility of those services. For several reasons, including higher per capita incomes and economies of scale in complementary health care inputs, there are many more physicians per capita in metropolitan areas than in non-metropolitan and rural areas.

III. Competition and the Market for Physicians Services

Provider network joint ventures have the potential to reduce costs and improve quality. Some physicians, however, have responded to changes in the market for physician services by engaging in collusive anticompetitive conduct, seeking collective bargaining rights, and manipulating licensure regulations. The following sections describe these developments and assess their implications for the cost, quality, and availability of health care. Some of these sections contain recommendations to enhance the performance of the physician services market.

A. Provider Network Joint Ventures

The Supreme Court's decisions in *Goldfarb* and*Maricopa* clarified the antitrust laws' application to health care, and spurred numerous market changes, including the development of managed care. Many physicians responded to managed care's growth by implementing network joint ventures to facilitate contracting with managed care plans. This section focuses on two joint venture types (IPAs and PHOs) and describes their key features and potential efficiencies. These joint venture types are not immutable categories; as managed care organizations (MCOs) have reduced reliance on capitation arrangements, some joint ventures have dissolved while others have implemented messenger models or invested in clinical integration. These joint ventures also compete with one another to recruit physician-members and to obtain MCO contracts.

1. IPAs

(a) Description of IPAs

IPAs are networks of independent physicians that contract with MCOs and employers. IPAs may be organized as sole proprietorships, partnerships, or professional corporations. Physician-members generally own IPAs, although individual doctors, hospitals or physician practice management companies also own some IPAs. IPAs contract with physicians on both an exclusive and nonexclusive basis. IPAs have historically included primary care physicians and specialists, although some commentators have noted a trend toward the formation of single-specialty IPAs. Many IPAs are nonprofit. IPAs can be integrated (financially, clinically, or both) to varying degrees or not at all. Physicians participating in financially integrated IPAs share financial risks. Clinically integrated IPAs seek to improve the quality of care their member-physicians provide though varied strategies. Physicians who eschew financially or clinically integrating an IPA may use a messenger model to convey price and price-related information to the payor.

Most IPAs emerged in the 1980s as a reaction to managed care. Panelists stated that some physicians in smaller practices thought that payors had the upper hand so they formed IPAs to gain bargaining leverage. Physicians were also concerned about missing out on managed care contracts, particularly contracts that included capitation provisions. One commentator stated that the Health Maintenance Organizations Act of 1973 spurred the growth of IP As by recognizing them as an acceptable form of organized medical practice and providing funds for their development. As MCOs have abandoned capitation arrangements with providers, the number of IP As has declined in recent years. Statistics on the number and size of IP As vary. A panelist representing an IPA trade association stated that there presently are approximately 2,000 IP As nationwide. One survey found that the number of IP As decreased from 1223 in 1996 to 771 in 2002. A national survey of physician organizations found that there were at least 463 IP As that contained more than 20 physician members in 2002.

One panelist noted that IP As can vary in size from about a dozen to more than 1,000 physician members. A national survey of physician organizations found the average number of doctors in an IPA was 233. Another study calculated an average of 387 physicians per IPA nationwide, while in California the average was 418.

(b) IPA Efficiencies

(i) Costs and Related Efficiencies: Panelists and commentators disagreed about the impact of IP As on the cost of care and whether IP As can create efficiencies. Panelists stated that IP As reduce contracting costs by lowering administrative and search costs for physicians and allowing payors to contract efficiently with pre-existing networks. Additionally, they asserted that IP As may generate efficiencies by integrating information technology and billing systems, using their collective purchasing power to receive volume discounts, and performing credentialing of physician-applicants.

Others expressed concern that physicians may use IPAs to obtain increased fees from payors. IPAs that engage in payor contracting and are not integrated run the risk of antitrust liability if they facilitate price agreements among their members. IPAs also create an additional layer of administration, which can increase administrative costs - although physician-members in the IPA have an incentive to minimize these expenses.

One panelist suggested that financial integration creates an incentive for physician-members to provide "quality care at the most cost effective price." Another panelist suggested that "pay for performance" (P4P) strategies, which are described in greater detail. A third panelist noted that P4P strategies have been adopted on an industry-wide basis in California. One study found that IPAs in California use 35-50 percent more care management strategies than physician organizations in other parts of the country. The study identified two factors that strongly correlated with this difference: IP As in California have greater exposure to external incentives to improve services and greater access to information technology than non-Californian IPAs. Panelists also considered whether clinical integration can reduce the cost of health care and create efficiencies. One panelist stated physicians in clinically integrated IP As can do a better job monitoring and managing patients with chronic illnesses. Such patients typically comprise five percent of the patient population but generate between 60 and 80 percent of health care costs. Another panelist stated that clinical integration allows physicians to share information more effectively. Two panelists reported that some IP As employ care management teams to coordinate patient care. On the other hand, commentators noted that clinical integration is very expensive, and cautioned that physicians may prove unwilling to make the necessary investment.

(ii) Quality of Care and Related Efficiencies: Some have stated that financial integration provides physicians with incentives to improve quality of care. Nevertheless, many physicians state that financial incentives including capitation arrangements reduce quality of care. One commentator observed that "[t]he degree to which capitation encourages organizations to compete on quality and efficiency depends on the market context within which it is used." Panelists stated that clinical integration can improve quality of care. One panelist observed that clinically integrated IPAs can "provide technology, clinical, and population management programs to improve patient care and outcomes." A capitated IPA that implemented certain clinical integration initiatives "exerted a dramatic impact on patterns of utilization and expenditure,"

noted one commentator. One study found that, although many IPAs have implemented organized care management programs to improve the quality of care for their patients, the use of such processes is still "relatively uncommon." Some experts contend that an integrated, or "closely knit" IPA may provide a good environment for testing whether quality programs can deliver hoped-for results.

2. PHOs

(a) Description of PHOs

A PHO is a joint venture between a hospital and physicians who generally have admitting privileges at the hospital. Physician and hospital members of a PHO sometimes contract jointly with MCOs for providing care to a population of patients. PHOs typically vary along four parameters: exclusivity, integration, ownership/control, and organizational base.

First, PHOs can accept hospital medical staff on an exclusive or nonexclusive basis. Open PHOs allow most medical staff to join and have minimum credentialing requirements; specialists usually dominate these PHOs. Closed PHOs limit physician membership by practice profiling or specialty type and are more likely to form exclusive relationships with physicians. PHOs that employ practice profiling seek to use objective practice data to determine which physicians they should invite to join the PHO. PHOs that recruit physician-members based on specialty type reportedly focus on the number of patients that the physician-member will see. Second, PHOs are integrated (whether financially, clinically, or both) to varying degrees or not at all. Many PHOs employ financial risk-sharing arrangements with physician-members, such as partial or full-risk contracts, although PHOs, as a whole, appear to be moving away from full-risk contracts. Third, ownership, control, and capital structure vary. Physician-members and hospitals jointly own most PHOs, but some hospitals are sole owners. Although hospitals generally provide a majority of initial capitalization, some PHOs strive for equal physician-hospital ownership. Physicians may own interests in a PHO individually or through an entity such as an IPA. PHOs can take the form of a limited liability company, a general partnership, a nonprofit corporation, or a general business corporation. Finally, PHOs can have different organizational bases. PHOs can have a hospital, multiple hospitals, or a hospital system as their organizational base. Commentators often describe PHOs that involve multiple hospitals or joint ventures between multiple PHOs as super-PHOs.

Panelists and commentators stated that PHOs emerged in the 1980s largely as "a defensive provider reaction to increasing managed care penetration." PHOs subsequently became the most common form of vertical integration among physicians and hospitals. Approximately 60 percent of PHOs are nonprofit and 40 percent are for-profit. In 2002, 74 percent of PHOs were open and 26 percent were closed. Panelists noted that PHOs have changed substantially in recent years. Many PHOs initially engaged in full or partial risk contracting. As insurers and providers abandoned capitated payment arrangements in favor of preferred provider organizations (PPOs) and point of service plans (POS plans), many PHOs scrambled to identify a new role to fill. Numerous PHOs have dissolved or failed in the last eight years. One antitrust lawyer panelist stated that his recent experience with PHOs primarily involves converting them into messenger model networks. PHOs that engage in payor contracting and are not integrated run the risk of antitrust liability if they facilitate price agreements among their members.

(b) PHO Efficiencies

(i) Costs and Related Efficiencies: Panelists and commentators differ on whether PHOs can reduce costs or otherwise result in efficiencies. Some contend that PHOs can reduce the cost of negotiating contracts between payors and physicians and hospitals by offering "one-stop shopping." As

such, PHOs may enable payors to contract more efficiently with physicians with whom they have no existing contractual arrangements. PHOs could also allow providers to contract directly with self-insured employers and certain Medicare and Medicaid risk or managed contracts. Commentators and panelists also stated that PHOs may deliver economies of scale by sharing administrative and integration costs among physician-members and hospitals. They further said that PHOs may result in more efficient deployment of physician resources, because these arrangements allow physician-members to concentrate on practicing medicine. Finally, they added that PHOs may reduce legal expenses for hospitals and physicians by enabling them to "present a unified front and a common defense in the event of malpractice claims." Others contend that the primary advantage for physicians and hospitals in forming a PHO is the increased bargaining power gained from "presenting a united front to payers." They assert that providers can use this additional bargaining power to obtain higher prices from payors, particularly if providers "raise barriers to entry by forming exclusive relationships." A panelist representing a health insurance plan stated that PHOs have given providers "greater negotiation leverage" and "contributed to some of the runaway inflation in health care costs." Empirical studies of PHO pricing have found mixed results. A recent study of hospital and physician integration based on organizations in Arizona, Florida, and Wisconsin found that integration is associated with an increase in prices, especially when the integrated organization is exclusive and located in less competitive markets. Other studies have concluded that physician-hospital affiliations generally do not result in higher hospital prices. Some commentators doubt whether PHOs actually lower the costs associated with contracting. One commentator stated that PHOs have not resulted "in any meaningful improvement in contracting ability. In many cases, MCOs already have provider contracts in place and see little value in going through the PHO."

(ii) Quality of Care and Related Efficiencies: Panelists and commentators differed on the ability of PHOs to improve quality of care. Some stated that PHOs can significantly improve quality by coordinating patient care delivered to consumers in the doctor's office and the hospital. They also stated that PHOs can implement shared information systems. One panelist representing a PHO contended that financially integrated PHOs can reduce costs and improve quality by clinically integrating. This panelist also suggested that physicians practicing individually or in small groups that are not financially or clinically integrated have limited ability to improve quality, reduce costs, and capture related efficiencies. The same panelist suggested that physicians practicing in large groups do not readily cooperate with one another, and hospitals are the most likely entities to implement programs to improve health care quality and reduce costs. Another panelist noted PHOs must make significant investments in clinical integration to improve quality of care. A third panelist suggested that clinical integration is improbable because of its high implementation costs and potential antitrust risks. A panelist representing a health insurance plan stated that "there appears to be no difference in the quality of care offered by a PHO than that offered by physicians and hospitals that contract separately." Although opinions regarding PHOs vary significantly, there is relatively little empirical research on PHOs, quality of care, and clinical integration with which to resolve these competing claims, and the available evidence is decidedly mixed.

3. Summary

Physicians have historically been solo or small-group practitioners, competing only with other such practitioners in their particular product and geographic market. As the market for physician services has evolved, and antitrust enforcement has addressed anticompetitive conduct, competition has emerged along multiple dimensions. IPAs and PHOs compete for physician-members and to contract with payors. The forms and modes of competition in the market for physician services will inevitably vary over time as conditions and preferences change. Competition helps deliver an optimum mix of physician services at the lowest cost and highest quality. The Agencies are committed to vigorous price and non-price competition and not to any particular model for delivering health care.

B. Physician Compensation

1. Physician Payment Arrangements

Insurers and others typically pay physicians on an FFS, salaried, or capitated basis. In FFS payment an insurer directly pays an individual provider based on the number and type of services that provider performs. Some state that FFS improves quality by rewarding physicians who do more for their patients. Other commentators are concerned that FFS payment creates incentives for physicians to over-provide healthcare resources because a physician's income is directly related to the volume and intensity of services rendered. Capitation involves a physician assuming responsibility for a certain number of patients and receiving a fixed amount for each of these patients regardless of whether those patients seek care. Although some state that capitation reduces the incentive to provide excessive care, others are concerned that capitation creates an incentive for physicians to increase the number of patients for whom they provide care and simultaneously decrease the services they actually provide.

Physicians employed by the government, hospitals, or medical groups typically receive a salary. Some commentators state that medical groups or organizations can align more carefully the incentives of the physician with those of the group by paying salaries. Others are concerned that such arrangements also create an incentive for physicians to decrease the number of patients they are responsible for and the services they provide. Medicare reimburses physicians on an FFS basis, using the resource-based relative value scale (RBRVS). The Centers for Medicare & Medicaid Services determine the RBRVS based on the cost of physician labor, practice overheads, materials, and liability insurance.

2. Messenger Model

a. Description of the Messenger Model: The messenger model is an arrangement that allows contracting between providers and payors, while avoiding price-fixing among competing providers. *Health Care Statement 9* provides that messenger models "can be organized and operated in a variety of ways." One panelist described the traditional messenger model as one involving a payor submitting fee schedules to an agent or third party, who transmits this schedule to the network physicians. This panelist elaborated that each physician decides individually whether to accept or reject the fee schedule and the messenger or agent communicates those decisions to the payor. The payor may then initiate another round of negotiations with the network physicians or enter into contracts with those physicians who accepted its offer, observed the panelist.

Commentators have discussed a variation that involves the messenger conveying to payors information obtained individually from providers about the prices or price-related terms that those providers are willing to accept. The messenger may aggregate this information into a comprehensive schedule and market the schedule to payors, and may receive authority from individual physicians to accept contractual offers on their behalf, commentators have noted. They also stated that agents must convey offers that do not meet a physician's preferred rate to those physicians, because they are not empowered to reject offers. Agents also may help physicians understand the contracts offered, for example, by providing objective or empirical information about the terms of an offer. Messenger models can be used creatively to facilitate contracting between payors and providers, so long as they do not facilitate anticompetitive agreements on price or other terms. Physician networks purporting to use the messenger model have given rise to considerable antitrust enforcement activity. In recent years, the Agencies have brought numerous cases alleging physicians involved in messenger models engaged in anticompetitive conduct. These cases have involved a diverse array of allegations.

b. Messenger Model Efficiencies and Antitrust Concerns: Panelists and commentators expressed differing views on whether the messenger model can reduce costs for providers and payors. Some stated that the messenger model simplifies contracting and contract administration, thereby reducing physicians' and payors' transaction costs. Two panelists observed that an agent can significantly reduce physicians' transaction costs by educating them about the terms of a contract. Panelists also explained that a properly implemented messenger model cannot result in higher prices for payors, because it is incapable of creating countervailing market power for physicians. Finally, one panelist observed that networks risk incurring administration costs for limited gain if only a minority of network physicians accept a payor's offer. In contrast, some panelists and commentators stated that the messenger model is not a viable business strategy and can increase costs for providers and payors. Panelists contended that such arrangements have high administrative costs because they are complex to implement and difficult to maintain. They observed that agents frequently cannot determine the antitrust implications of a particular course of conduct and therefore require expensive legal advice. Others noted that certain messenger model variations actually can prolong contract negotiations and increase provider and payor transaction costs.

Panelists and commentators also differed on the messenger model's usefulness in avoiding antitrust concerns. Some stated that messenger arrangements are useful in preventing violations of the antitrust laws and lower the risk of being compelled to disband a network to settle an Agency investigation. One panelist noted the model has been particularly useful for erstwhile financially integrated physician networks that need an alternative contracting mechanism as risk sharing arrangements have become less common. Others noted that physician networks purporting to use the messenger model have been the focus of multiple Agency investigations and consent settlements.

3. Physician Collective Bargaining

Some physicians have lobbied heavily for statutory or other legal changes that would enable independent physicians to bargain collectively by exempting them from the antitrust laws. Those who support such exemptions contend that physicians need to bargain collectively to exercise countervailing market power against payors. The Agencies have consistently opposed such exemptions because they are likely to harm consumers by increasing costs without improving quality of care. This section describes the legal landscape for physician collective bargaining, discusses the competitive impact of countervailing power, and considers the impact of collective bargaining on the cost and quality of health care.

(a) Legal Landscape: Both labor and antitrust laws affect the ability of workers to bargain collectively. Antitrust law prohibits competitors from price-fixing and engaging in group boycotts. Labor law provides exemptions from antitrust liability under certain circumstances. Pursuant to the National Labor Relations Act (NLRA), employed physicians are generally allowed to unionize and bargain collectively. Physicians who are self-employed or independent contractors generally may not collectively bargain without violating the antitrust laws. A few states have passed legislation that exempts self-employed physicians from the antitrust laws and provides for state regulation of physician collective bargaining. Other states and Congress have also considered such legislation. Commission staff submitted competition advocacy letters commenting on three such bills in Ohio, Washington, and Alaska.

Until recently, physician interest in unionization and collective bargaining was limited. Organized medicine long opposed physician unions. According to one panelist, physicians began making more concerted efforts to unionize and bargain collectively in the 1970's in response to the emergence of large health care organizations and changes in physician fees. The same panelist noted that many physicians believed that organized medicine was failing to respond to these changes. The AMA remained opposed to unionization until 1999 when it approved the formation of Physicians for Responsible Negotiations (PRN). Initially, PRN was "an AMA-affiliated labor organization dedicated to representing physicians in collective bargaining with employers." Panelists primarily attributed the AMA's support for physician unionization to an ongoing decline in the AMA's total membership and a determined lobbying effort by the AMA's younger physician members. News reports indicate that PRN's membership in 2002 was "only a few hundred" individual members, its advocacy for two Chicago physicians' groups had stalled, and that "AMA leaders, who fear that union-management tensions would compromise patient care, ha[ve] stymied the group." In March 2004, the AMA and PRN separated; PRN now operates as an independent physician labor organization.

(b) Countervailing Power: Some physicians claim they need countervailing market power to offset the market power they allege health care insurers possess. They contend that monopsony power enables health plans to approach "contract negotiations with a 'take-it-or-leave-it' attitude that puts physicians in the untenable position of accepting inappropriate contract terms." The AMA asserts that these terms include unreasonably low fees and provisions that may harm quality of care. Some participants asserted that there are numerous markets in which health care insurers exercise monopsony power. Others disagreed, however, arguing that physicians, rather than insurers, often exercise market power. Although there may be disparities in bargaining position between some payors and some providers, the available evidence does not

indicate that there is a monopsony power problem in most health care markets.

A proponent of countervailing power theory stated that providers need this power if health care insurers exercise monopsony power. Nonetheless, those physicians seeking to bargain collectively have sought blanket exemptions from the antitrust laws. Several speakers opposed such exemptions. As one panelist stated, "it's clear that a blanket exemption to the antitrust laws for the purpose of allowing the creation of countervailing power is inappropriate." Another speaker similarly testified that allowing providers to acquire countervailing market power is unnecessary, impossible to implement, and bad public policy.

The Agencies believe that antitrust enforcement to prevent the unlawful acquisition or exercise of monopsony power by insurers is a better solution than allowing providers to exercise countervailing power. Joel Klein, the Assistant Attorney General in 1999, noted that a "better approach [than allowing countervailing market power] is to empower consumers by encouraging price competition, opening the flow of accurate, meaningful information to consumers, and ensuring effective antitrust enforcement both with regard to buyers (health care insurance plans) and sellers (health care professionals) of provider services." Former FTC Chairman Robert Pitofsky likewise remarked that "[f]rom a policy and enforcement perspective, the most effective response to the emergence of excessive buyer power is not to permit the aggregation of some form of countervailing power. Rather, the appropriate response is to try to prevent the aggregation of excessive buying power in the first place."

Panelists agreed that it is preferable to use antitrust enforcement to address monopsony concerns than to allow physicians to accumulate countervailing market power. One panelist stated, for example, that the best policy response to the existence of market power on one side of the market is to remove it on a case-by-case basis. Even a panelist who spoke in favor of allowing countervailing market power noted that restoring competition is the ideal solution to a health insurer's acquisition of monopsony power.

Indeed, even if we assume physicians confront a monopsonist health plan that neither unlawfully acquired nor unlawfully exercised that power, authorizing physicians to engage in collusive conduct will not serve the interests of consumers. A health insurer with monopsony power is likely to impose quantity restrictions that will increase prices for consumers. If providers were to acquire countervailing market power, the result is likely to be further quantity restrictions - increasing the prices paid by consumers above those already imposed by the monopsonist.

Providers that obtain countervailing market power also likely will cause competitive harm to other market participants that do not possess monopsony power. One panelist suggested, for example, that physicians may use their countervailing market power to disadvantage non-physician competitors, such as nurse midwives and nurse anesthetists, or health care insurers other than the monopsonist health care insurer. The Agencies believe that statutory or other legal changes allowing countervailing market power are ill-advised and unnecessary. To the extent monopsony power exists in some markets, the Agencies and state Attorneys General should address such matters on a case-by-case basis.

(c) Physician Collective Bargaining Harms Consumers: The Agencies have consistently opposed the creation of antitrust exemptions for physician collective bargaining. In congressional testimony, the Agencies have identified various ways in which physician collective bargaining likely will harm consumers and other participants in the health care system.

These harms include: (i) consumers and employers facing higher prices for health insurance coverage; (ii) consumers facing higher out-of-pocket expenses as copayments and other unreimbursed expenses increase; (iii) consumers receiving reduced benefits as costs increase; (iv) senior citizens participating in Medicare HMOs receiving reduced benefits; (v) the federal government paying more for health coverage for its employees; (vi) state and local governments incurring higher costs to provide health benefits to their employees; (vii) state Medicaid programs incurring higher costs to provide health benefits, forcing them to increase taxes, cut benefits, or reduce the number of beneficiaries; and (viii) the number of uninsured increasing due to more costly health insurance. The balance of this section focuses on the impact of physician collective bargaining on cost and quality. Collective bargaining is likely to increase substantially the price of health care services, because providers collectively are likely to demand higher fees and refuse to negotiate individually. The Agencies have extensive experience with the consequences of alleged physician collective bargaining. For example, the Commission alleged approximately 500 physicians and 15 hospitals that comprised the vast majority of providers covering a large area of southern Georgia conspired to fix prices and not to deal with payors on an individual basis. According to the complaint, respondents restrained competition among the providers and forced payors to pay higher prices to its providers, thereby increasing the cost of healthcare for consumers.

In *United States v. Federation of Physicians And Dentists,* the Division alleged that the Federation had successfully recruited virtually all of the private practice orthopedic surgeons in Delaware, who ultimately agreed to designate the Federation as their exclusive agent to negotiate fee levels with a particular payor. The Federation then organized nearly all of its members to terminate their contracts with this payor with the expectation that this would force that payor to accede to their fee demands. There are many other examples of such conduct.

The Congressional Budget Office (CBO) estimated that proposed federal legislation to exempt physicians from antitrust scrutiny and allow collective bargaining "would increase expenditures on private health insurance by 2.6 percent." The CBO also predicted that such legislation would increase direct federal spending on healthcare programs such as Medicaid by $11.3 billion and decrease tax revenue by $10.9 billion over ten years. Other estimates of the cost of an antitrust waiver were substantially higher. Physician groups have argued that the actual cost of physician collective bargaining is likely to be modest. Whatever the impact on costs, proponents of antitrust exemptions for physicians often suggest that collective bargaining will result in increased quality of care. However, physician collective bargaining has historically focused on physician compensation and not on patient care issues. Moreover, as explains in this chapter, current antitrust law already permits physicians to work collectively on legitimate quality of care issues. Given these considerations, physician collective bargaining is unlikely to improve the quality of care that consumers receive.

C. Licensure, Market Entry, and Practice Restrictions

Licensure impacts marketplace competition. Through licensure requirements, states may restrict market entry by physicians and allied health professionals (AHPs), and further limit the scope of authorized practice. Most state licensing boards are primarily composed of licensed providers, although some states require broader representation. The Commission recently initiated administrative litigation against a state licensing board, alleging that it had taken steps unlawfully to restrict AHPs from obtaining direct access to consumers. Many states have only limited or no reciprocity for licensing out-of-state physicians and AHPs seeking to practice in-state. A number of state licensing boards have also sought to restrict the practice of telemedicine. This section considers each of these issues and recommends strategies for addressing the anticompetitive risks of state regulation of the nature and form of professional practice.

1. Mechanisms to Regulate Physician and AHP Market Entry

The states have traditionally assumed responsibility for regulating physicians and AHPs using three distinct mechanisms: (i) occupational licensing or licensure; (ii) certification; and (iii) registration. Licensure, the most restrictive method of regulation, typically involves a mandatory system of state-imposed standards that practitioners must meet to practice a given profession. Autonomous boards, comprised largely of members of the regulated profession, determine applicants' eligibility requirements, develop standards of practice, and enforce disciplinary actions. Physicians and other licensed professionals must satisfy these requirements to practice within the state. Certification generally refers to a voluntary system of standards that practitioners can choose to meet to demonstrate accomplishment or ability in their profession. Nongovernmental agencies or associations typically set certification standards. Certified health professionals may use a predetermined title. Uncertified health professionals may still practice within the field but may not use the relevant title. Certification can serve as a substitute for and a complement to licensure. Many physicians become board certified within a specialty, in order to establish that they have an appropriate level of knowledge, skills, and experience.

Registration is the least restrictive mechanism for regulating health care professionals because individuals simply must file their name, address, and qualifications with a government agency to practice. Professionals generally are not required to meet educational or experience requirements to practice under a registration system.

(a) Regulation's Impact on Cost, Quality, and Access: Commentators state that limits on entry increase health care costs. However, commentators and panelists disagreed on the effects of licensing on quality of care. Several commentators contend that a state-enforced minimum quality standard is

an efficient response to the "limited information patients have about quality and the relatively high costs of obtaining information." Another commentator noted that "[o]ccupational licensure creates a greater incentive for individuals to invest in more occupation-specific human capital because they will be more able to recoup the full returns to their investment if they need not face low-quality substitutes for their services." Others argue that licensure may not improve quality of care because the requirements do not correspond to the factors that influence quality. Moreover, some maintain that licensure may decrease the overall quality of care that consumers receive by increasing prices, which can cause some consumers to forego care.

Empirical studies have found that licensing regulation increases costs for consumers. There are fewer studies on the impact of licensure on quality, and these studies have found mixed results. One study found that licensure requirements can reduce the likelihood of adverse outcomes and increase quality of care. Another study found that consumers in states with tougher licensure requirements do not receive higher quality care, because the resulting increase in the price of care limits consumer access. A third study found that licensure benefits the segment of consumers who place more emphasis on quality. Studies consistently have found that state-based licensure can harm consumer welfare by serving as a barrier to provider mobility.

(b) Certification's Impact on Cost, Quality, and Access: Some commentators state that certification, rather than licensure, is a better way to protect quality, increase consumer choice, broaden access to care, and enhance market competition. They state that providing consumers with a choice of certified or uncertified providers allows consumers to receive care they might forego under a licensure regime. Some commentators also contend that certification spurs competition and innovation by creating increased opportunities for market entry.

Others argue, however, that certification does not adequately protect consumers from low quality care and suggest that consumers may not factor in certain externalities when they select uncertified health care providers. Moreover, if health plans only choose to cover certified health care providers, a certification regime may not markedly increase the choices available to consumers. There currently is insufficient empirical evidence to assess whether certification provides many of the benefits of licensure with fewer disadvantages. The Agencies encourage further study of the advantages and disadvantages of these two methods for regulating physician and AHP market entry.

2. AHPs and Provider Control of Licensure Boards

Most state statutes delegate authority for establishing and enforcing licensure standards to state Boards of Medical Examiners. These boards typically promulgate regulations governing physicians and related AHPs. Because most board members are industry participants with economic interests at stake, the potential exists for the board to make decisions that are contrary to consumers' interests. Panelists and commentators have identified varying ways in which provider-controlled state-based licensure boards can limit competition and harm consumers. A panelist representing a dental hygienists' trade association described the efforts of certain Boards of Dentistry to prevent dental hygienists from obtaining direct access to consumers. This panelist stated that such Boards determinedly seek to maintain control over dental hygienists and contended that this control denies consumers access to dental care. This panelist also asserted that the Boards of Dentistry in certain states have prevented dental hygienists from obtaining direct payment, despite those states' Departments of Health authorizing such hygienists to provide certain services to consumers without a dentist's supervision. These arrangements, argued the panelist, increase dental costs and decrease consumers' access to dental care.

The Commission recently alleged the South Carolina State Board of Dentistry "restrained competition in the provision of preventive dental care services by unreasonably restricting the delivery of dental cleanings, sealants, and topical fluoride treatments in school settings by licensed dental hygienists." The Board contends that its challenged actions were necessary to protect school children from substandard care, including possible injury. Many commentators state that widening the membership of state licensure boards will decrease the probability that provider-dominated licensure boards will harm competition. The Institute of Medicine (IOM) recommended that "states strengthen the accountability and broaden the public base of their regulatory statutes and procedures." In particular, the IOM recommended that "[l]icensing boards should draw at least half of their membership from outside the licensed occupation; members should be drawn from the public as well as from a variety of areas of expertise such as health administration, economics, consumer affairs, education, and health services research." States should consider adopting the IOM's recommendation to expand the membership of state licensure boards. Such reform may reduce the possibility that these boards will engage in conduct that increases prices or decreases access to health care.

3. State Restrictions on the Interstate Practice of Telemedicine

Interstate communications between health professionals historically have not been subject to licensing requirements. As the Department of Health and Human Services (HHS) noted, "the consulted physician or other health professional [was] regarded either as practicing medicine only in his or her home state or as exempt from licensure under the 'consultation exception' in the patient's state." Developments in technology have facilitated the practice of telemedicine, which involves the use of electronic communication and information technologies to provide or support clinical care at a distance. Telemedicine can benefit consumers in at least three ways. First, telemedicine can give physicians and other health care professionals the ability to provide high quality medical services to rural or other underserved areas.

Second, telemedicine can significantly reduce a range of health-care-related costs, including travel expenses and costs arising from the duplication of services, technologies, and specialists. With telemedicine, for example, a single pathologist can provide services to a number of locations. Finally, telemedicine networks can enhance training and education in new technologies for health care professionals, particularly for those located in rural areas. After surveying empirical studies on the costs and benefits of telemedicine, HHS observed "there may be real cost savings to be realized from telemedicine."

Telemedicine can harm consumers in at least four ways. First, telemedicine can subject consumers to substandard care, possibly from unlicensed providers. Individual states have a legitimate interest in ensuring that out-of-state health professionals meet the same standards as professionals licensed within the state. Second, providers could use telemedicine to perpetrate fraud against consumers. Third, "[t]elemedicine consultations might involve personal medical records being shipped over computer lines to other regions of the country," creating privacy and confidentiality concerns. Finally, "[t]here is significant uncertainty regarding whether malpractice insurance policies cover services provided by telemedicine."

The practice of telemedicine has thus crystallized tensions between the states' role in ensuring patients have access to quality care and the anticompetitive effects of protecting in-state physicians from out-of-state competition. Many states have responded to telemedicine by enacting legislation to restrict such practices. HHS reported that 11 states had implemented laws restricting the interstate practice of telemedicine in 1997, and 26 states had implemented such laws by 2001. These states mostly require a physician to obtain either a special license to engage in the out-of-state practice of medicine or a full unrestricted state medical license.

Some contend these laws may create a barrier to entry that significantly increases costs and decreases access without improving quality of care for physicians who want to practice telemedicine.

Commentators have debated varied approaches to encourage the practice of telemedicine. Some have argued that Congress should pass national telemedicine licensure laws to stop individual states from protecting the economic interests of their providers to the detriment of their citizens' access to healthcare. Others contend that telemedicine should be regulated on a state-by-state basis. The American Telemedicine Association (ATA) has proposed an alternative, which it argues is "a compromise between full national licensure and state-imposed unreasonable barriers" to telemedicine. The ATA contends that states should regulate physical face-to-face encounters between physicians and patients within state borders, but not virtual consultations across state borders. They also recommend that states should not restrict a duly licensed physician from consulting a physician in another state.

When used properly, telemedicine has considerable promise as a mechanism to broaden access, lower costs, and increase healthcare quality. When used improperly, telemedicine has the potential to lower health care quality and increase the incidence of consumer fraud. To foster telemedicine's likely pro-competitive benefits and to deter its potential to harm consumers, states should consider implementing uniform licensure standards or reciprocity compacts. Uniform licensure standards and reciprocity compacts could operate both to protect consumers and to reduce barriers to telemedicine. State regulators and legislators should explicitly consider the pro-competitive benefits of telemedicine before restricting it.

IV. Antitrust Enforcement in the Physician Marketplace

This section examines the application of competition law to the marketplace for physician services. It first discusses the significance of private antitrust litigation involving physician privileges and credentialing. The section then discusses the Agencies' analysis of provider network joint ventures, focusing on market developments in financial and clinical integration. Finally, this section addresses the ability of physicians to share and use quality-related information and the application of the state action doctrine to licensure and physician collective bargaining.

A. Private Litigation Involving Physician Privileges and Credentialing

The most common type of private healthcare-related antitrust litigation raises physician privilege or credentialing issues. These cases usually involve physicians asserting that a hospital and/or its physician peer review committee denied them privileges for anticompetitive reasons. Physicians with hospital privileges may also sue hospitals and/or their peer review committee because these privileges have been revoked or curtailed. Commentators state that the courts largely have been "inhospitable" to these cases, except when there has been "clear evidence of bad faith by rival physicians on the hospital's medical staff[, which has] resulted in large damage awards." An empirical study found that plaintiff physicians prevail in only seven percent of these cases. One set of commentators are concerned, however, that these "staff privileges cases have had problematic effects on the legal analysis of quality-based competition" because the "courts began using quality to remove conduct from the purview of competition law, rather than factoring quality into an overall competitive mix." Congress created an antitrust safe harbor for peer review decisions involving quality that meet certain procedural requirements in the *Health Care Quality Improvement Act of 1986*. This legislation also enabled prevailing defendants to seek recovery of attorney's fees. The number of physician privilege antitrust cases dropped by approximately 10 percent in the decade following the passage of this Act.

B. Provider Network Joint Ventures

The antitrust analysis of joint ventures and multi-provider networks has received considerable attention from the Agencies and commentators in recent years. This issue is not unique to health care; as the Commission recently stated, "no analytical exercise is more important to U.S. competition policy than defining the bounds of acceptable cooperation between direct rivals." As noted previously, the Agencies have brought numerous enforcement actions against physician networks, and also issued statements, advisory opinions, and business review letters on this subject.

1. The Agencies' Antitrust Analysis of Provider Network Joint Ventures

Health Care Statement 8 describes how the Agencies evaluate physician network joint ventures. This statement sets forth antitrust safety zones for exclusive and non-exclusive physician network joint ventures that, absent extraordinary circumstances, the Agencies are unlikely to challenge. *Statement* 8 then outlines the analytical framework for joint ventures that fall outside the antitrust safety zones. It states that like transactions in other sectors of the economy, "physician network joint ventures will be analyzed under the rule of reason, and will not be viewed as per se illegal, if the physicians' integration through the network is likely to produce significant efficiencies that benefit consumers, and any price agreements (or other agreements that would otherwise be per se illegal) by the network physicians are reasonably necessary to realize those efficiencies."

This statement further notes that financial risk-sharing and clinical integration may involve sufficient integration to demonstrate that the venture is likely to produce significant efficiencies. Finally, *Statement* 8 outlines the Agencies' rule of reason analytical framework and applies the principles set forth in the statement to seven examples of physician network joint ventures.

2. Financial Integration

Statement 8 notes that financial risk sharing can generate significant efficiencies by providing physicians with incentives to cooperate in controlling the cost and improving the quality of services they render. It provides examples of arrangements through which participants in a physician network joint venture can share substantial financial risk, including capitation, global fee arrangements, fee-withholds, and cost or utilization-based bonuses or penalties. *Statement* 8 also establishes that only those physician networks that share substantial financial risk can qualify for an antitrust safety zone on the basis of their financial integration.

The *Health Care Statements* acknowledge, financing and delivery arrangements for health care have changed substantially over the past several decades. Some commentators and panelists state P4P arrangements may have important procompetitive benefits for consumers. In determining whether a physician network joint venture is sufficiently financially integrated to warrant rule of reason analysis, the Agencies will consider the extent to which a particular P4P arrangement constitutes the sharing of substantial financial risk among the members of the joint venture, whether that sharing is likely to produce efficiencies, and whether any price or otherwise per se illegal agreements among the members are reasonably necessary to achieve those efficiencies.

3. Clinical Integration

Health Care Statement 8 notes that clinical integration can be evidenced by a "network implementing an active and ongoing program to evaluate and modify practice patterns by the network's physician participants and create a high degree of interdependence and cooperation among the physicians to control costs and ensure quality." This statement identifies three arrangements that a clinical integration program might include: (i) establishing mechanisms to monitor and control utilization of health care services that are designed to control costs and assure quality of care; (ii) selectively choosing network physicians who are likely to further these efficiency objectives; and (iii) the significant investment of capital, both monetary and human, in the necessary infrastructure and capability to realize the claimed efficiencies.

This section discusses commentators' perspectives on clinical integration and presents a series of inquiries the Agencies are likely to pose when considering whether a physician network joint venture is sufficiently clinically integrated to avoid summary condemnation. Commission staff stated in an advisory opinion to a proposed initiative involving clinical integration that the venture, as designed, did not warrant summary condemnation. Commission staff also closed an investigation into a physician collaboration that created a substantial degree of market concentration, because the parties demonstrated the collaboration created considerable efficiencies (including improvements in the quality of care).

(a) Indicia of Clinical Integration: Commentators and industry experts describe various techniques and programs for achieving clinical integration. Commentators primarily focus on four indicia of clinical integration: (1) the use of common information technology to ensure exchange of all relevant patient data; (2) the development and adoption of clinical protocols; (3) care review based on the implementation of protocols; and (4) mechanisms to ensure adherence to protocols. Panelists and industry experts also have discussed other indicia of clinical integration including physician credentialing, case management, preauthorization of medical care, and review of associated hospital stays. Some also have discussed the use of payment systems to collect clinical data.

Commentators described varied information technology (IT) systems that can facilitate, monitor, and control the utilization of health care services. The FTC MedSouth Letter discussed, for example, an IT system that included "a web-based electronic clinical data record system that will permit MedSouth physicians to access and share clinical information relating to their patients."

Some suggest that these systems can significantly improve quality of care by enabling physicians to collect and track information about individual patients. One industry expert noted the "management of information as it relates to promoting health, treating illness and managing disease" is a "major component of clinical integration." Some have observed that clinical care information technology systems are expensive to implement. One study found that California-based IPAs are among the most successful in implementing and using IT systems, in part because they employ more technical support staff.

Commentators describe physicians' selection and adoption of care management protocols (CMPs) as another indicia of clinical integration. A trade association representing Californian physician groups stated that these protocols can "delineate utilization and quality goals for various diagnoses." This trade association also described the process by which an IPA might develop and revise clinical protocols. MedSouth proposed to implement between 100 and 150 such protocols that would cover 80-90 percent of the diagnoses that were prevalent in their physician members' practices. Commentators have observed that the selection and implementation of CMPs can improve quality and generate efficiencies for physician networks and payors. Several commentators contend, however, that clinical integration requires networks to monitor and ensure compliance with CMPs.

(b) Are Joint Negotiations on Price Reasonably Necessary to Achieve Clinical Integration? A joint venture will escape summary condemnation when joint price negotiations are reasonably necessary to achieve substantial efficiencies arising from the clinical integration. Panelists and commentators identified varying reasons why joint negotiations may be

reasonably necessary to implement and maintain a clinical integration program.

A trade association representing Californian physician groups contended that joint negotiation of contracts will ensure that sufficient physicians across multiple specialties participate in the venture. Physicians participate in IPA networks, this association argued, because they can delegate "the time and hassle of negotiating contracts with payers" to the IPA. Moreover, the trade association suggested that payors' overall costs may not necessarily increase, because a clinically integrated IPA will deliver cost-effective and efficient care. This trade association also argued that clinically integrated IPAs "can offer payers a single, comprehensive, and integrated network" and should therefore "be priced in the aggregate, not through individual contracts with physicians."

Commentators similarly asserted that joint pricing is necessary to ensure the active and ongoing participation of an entire group's members. These commentators also contend that joint negotiations are necessary to help physician members recover the substantial time and financial commitments that are necessary to implement a clinical integration program. Finally, they argue that joint negotiations are necessary to prevent physician members from free-riding on the contributions of their colleagues. The extent to which joint contracting is reasonably necessary to achieve efficient clinical integration will vary, depending on the facts and circumstances. The Agencies will consider multiple factors to determine whether collective negotiation is reasonably necessary to accomplish the goal of achieving clinical integration. Participants in a joint venture that is not sufficiently integrated (whether financially or clinically) face significant antitrust risk if they attempt to contract jointly.

(c) Further Guidance on Clinical Integration: Commentators and panelists asserted that there is uncertainty regarding the nature and extent of clinical integration that would, in

the Agencies' view, avoid summary condemnation of collective price setting or other horizontal agreements on competitive terms among physicians who participate in clinically integrated joint ventures. Several panelists and commentators requested that the Agencies provide additional guidance to address such uncertainty. The Agencies are committed to eliminating unlawful restraints on vigorous price and non-price competition in physician markets, but not to any particular model for financing and delivering health care. The Agencies do not suggest particular structures with which to achieve clinical integration that justifies joint pricing, because it would risk channeling market behavior rather than encouraging market participants to develop structures responsive to their particular efficiency goals and the market conditions they favor.

Nonetheless, to help further guide practitioners and counsel on the issue, below is a broad outline of some of the kinds of questions that the Agencies are likely to ask when analyzing the competitive implications of a physician network joint venture that justifies joint action involving price or other competitively significant terms on the grounds that it is clinically integrated. The Agencies emphasize that this list is not exhaustive, and that these questions may be more or less relevant, depending on factual circumstances. Other questions, not listed here, may be important, again depending on the facts at issue.

1. What do the physicians plan to do together from a clinical standpoint?
   - What specific activities will (and should) be undertaken?
   - How does this differ from what each physician already does individually?
   - What ends are these collective activities designed to achieve?
2. How do the physicians expect actually to accomplish these goals?
   - What infrastructure and investment is needed?

- What specific mechanisms will be put in place to make the program work?
- What specific measures will there be to determine whether the program is in fact working?

3. What basis is there to think that the individual physicians will actually attempt to accomplish these goals?
   - How are individual incentives being changed and re-aligned?
   - What specific mechanisms will be used to change and re-align the individual incentives?
4. What results can reasonably be expected from undertaking these goals?
   - Is there any evidence to support these expectations, in terms of empirical support from the literature or actual experience?
   - To what extent is the potential for success related to the group's size and range of specialities?
5. How does joint contracting with payors contribute to accomplishing the program's clinical goals?
   - Is joint pricing reasonably necessary to accomplish the goals?
   - In what ways?
6. To accomplish the group's goals, is it necessary (or desirable) for physicians to affiliate exclusively with one IPA or can they effectively participate in multiple entities and continue to contract outside the group?
   - Why or why not?

C. Physician Information Sharing

The sharing of information among physicians can have procompetitive benefits, but may also facilitate collusion or otherwise reduce competition on prices or compensation. *Health Care Statement* 6 sets forth a safety zone for provider exchange of price and cost information that the Agencies will not challenge, absent extraordinary circumstances. The statement also outlines the Agencies' antitrust analysis of information exchanges that fall outside this safety zone. The Agencies have issued a number of business review letters and advisory opinions that apply the analytical framework in *Statement* 6 to evaluate the antitrust implications of physicians' collecting and disseminating information concerning insurer payments for physician services. In general, the sharing of quality-related information among physicians and consumers can reduce costs and increase quality of care. As Areeda and Hovenkamp note, "the great majority of exchanges of information that do not pertain to either price or output should be regarded as harmless, at least when concerted refusals to deal are not in issue." The Agencies encourage such information sharing, as long as there are adequate safeguards to ensure information exchange is not used for anticompetitive ends.

Index